THE HEALTHIER GREEK

TAKE CONTROL OF YOUR INSULIN RESISTANCE OR DIABETES WHILE EATING GREAT TASTING FOOD!

By Demme Matheos, AADP

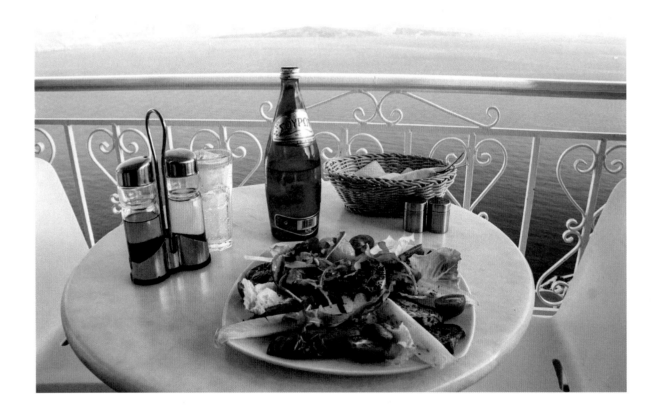

Dedication

This Book is dedicated to my beautiful, loving, smart and amazing mother Eugenia Matheos who instilled in me the love of Greek cooking and culture in the short 15½ years I had with her. I love you mom and I thank you for everything you have taught me in that short amazing time. The memories are in my heart forever.

This book is also dedicated to all the beautiful strong women that have passed through my lifetime so far. You have all made me who I am today and I thank you from the bottom of my heart for every loving gesture, remark, and lesson...

Tina Muller who continued where my mom left off and watched over us like a second mom.

Violet Azarian gave us love and attention and showed us how to have fun and enjoy every little thing without using money.

Gia Gia Anna Matheos you watched us every summer and pushed us to be strong, independent women and not take anything lying down.

Bahia Mokhtar Attia I miss your laugh and love of your family. Thank you for showing me what that looks like. I know how hard you worked to keep everyone together and I love you and miss you.

Stella Matheos thank you for sharing your love of cooking and your mom Gia Gia Ermioni Koffinas with me. The kindness and strength that comes out of this woman is just jaw dropping.

Nina Sarris thanks for showing me what the words kindness, good heartedness, and strong look like. I love being part of your family and I appreciate you always remembering my son on every holiday and treating him like a grandson.

This book is also dedicated to two amazing Doctors who have changed my life forever. They have been persistent in their teachings and fully dedicated in getting the world healthier one person at a time. This is also my goal. I feel it is my calling in life to help people get healthier by sharing my story.

Dr. David Wendell, owner and founder of Health and Wellness Center in Jackson, NJ, whom I met in the beginning of my journey back in 2007. Dr. George Kosmides who made a huge impact on my life in such a short time. I thank you both for all your knowledge and I will forever remember your words. You both have helped me become the person I am today through just being you and showing up as amazing human beings on a daily basis.

TABLE OF CONTENTS

Dedication

Foreword

Thank You

Introduction

Foreword

I am Dr. Dave Wendel, a practicing doctor of chiropractic for almost 30 years and director of the Natural Health & Wellness Center, a functional wellness facility, located in downtown Jamesburg, NJ. Our facility specializes in helping people regain their health through lifestyle modification, specializing in nutrition, and dietary support as a way to overcome *dis-ease*.

I first met Demme Matheos back in 2010, when she came to my office seeking help and guidance in order to regain her health. Initially Demme struggled for results with our program and guidance, allowing not only the influences of the world, but also the influences of her family, to control her life. Her health ended up spiraling out of control. I was able to have a conversation with her in early 2011 regarding the bleak potential for her future. I asked Demme whether or not she wanted to be a participating member in her son's life? This point truly hit home for her. Realizing that there could be a good chance that she would miss out watching her son grow up, she made the firm decision, and then had the determination, not only to significantly improve upon her health but to learn how she could help others improve upon their health as well.

Since that conversation, Demme has committed to becoming healthier. When I first started treating her she was dealing with chronic fatigue, a brittle stiff body, and an ashen appearance. She has blossomed into a person full of energy, flexibility, and a great natural complexion. Demme's book is one that she has amassed over the past several years as she has transformed herself and learned about health, that which is truly healthy and not the rhetoric spewed on television or over the internet. She has also recorded her progress.

The area that stands out the most for me concerning Demme is her endearment to the knowledge of healthy eating. As with most people who enter our office, learning how to eat healthy is a process. Demme, over the past several years, has made it her mission to not only develop good eating habits, but more importantly has learned how to transform classic Greek dishes into healthier options in order to feed her family. Now she desires to share her knowledge and practical experience with the world. This is her way to give back to mankind for all the blessings she has been bestowed.

I am truly honored to be writing this foreword for *The Healthier Greek* and honored to be a part of Demme's world, sharing what truly matters to her, health and wellness. She also loves to share with others so that they too may unlock their full potential while excelling and living life to the fullest!

Enjoy the book, take time to experience the dishes that are recorded within its pages. Use the time making these meals to nourish both your family's bodies and minds. Consider cooking some of these meals together, sharing in the process, and deepening your relationships.

Well done Demme!

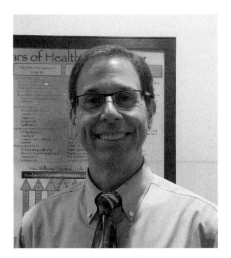

Dr. Dave Wendel

Thank you for helping!

A portion of the proceeds from the purchase of this book will be going to organizations helping those dealing with diseases and conditions that my mother suffered with throughout her short life.

Introduction

It all started on Mother's Day, 2010. I felt like I was having a heart attack!!

My heart was racing. My arm was tense. I remember those feelings to this day. It took me hours to decide to finally get in the car and drive to the Emergency Room. I made the decision for my son who was 6 years old at the time. He was and is my life. I didn't want him to be worried, sad or scared, and I also didn't want to DIE!!

So I got in the car and drove to the Emergency Room. The Doctor came in, asked a few questions, and said, "Are you trying to kill yourself?

Do you understand how you will die if you don't take care of your health?"

My son was in the room and heard all of this!! It was the worse day of my life to see my son start crying and listen to him screaming, "Mommy NO, please don't die, please don't die!"

That is when they put me in the hospital for further testing. Thank God I wasn't having a heart attack. I was diagnosed with Angina and so many other issues. High cholesterol, anxiety, diabetes, high blood pressure, and Chronic Obstructive Pulmonary Disease or COPD (a lung disease).

I WAS SCARED!!

How did I get here? I knew I had felt 'off' for the past few months and hadn't made myself a priority.

I thought, I don't want to die! I must do something about it NOW!!

Once I was released from the hospital, I started making a few simple changes and things started getting better.

Throughout my life I have been on so many diets, too many to count. The one thing they all had in common was dry bland BORING foods. I knew I wouldn't be able to stick to any of them for a lifetime, especially if the food didn't taste good.

I also knew I had to make a lifestyle change and I had to make it doable for my entire family.

I don't want another generation of my family having to deal with these symptoms or end up with diabetes, obesity, heart disease, anxiety, depression, infertility issues, leaky gut, etc.

I especially don't want our beautiful son to ever have to go through what I went through in my lifetime. I want this 'dis-ease' to stop here with me!!

For the past 4 years I have made an effort to not put weight loss as my focus. I teach that to my clients as well. Focusing on bio-individuality is the key.

Now I am down 75 pounds from a tight size 28 to size 18/20. In fact the week before I ended up in the hospital I had bought a size 32 blouse. It was a horrible feeling knowing that I kept getting bigger and bigger and didn't try to do anything about it!!

After years of cleaning up all the damage I have finally gotten rid of my diabetes medications via eating healthy, moving more, and working on how I react to stress in my life. I still have another 55 pounds to lose in order to do skin surgery. I know I will reach it and never turn back.

Each day I am learning new habits and seeing what works for me in my life.

This book has been on my mind for a few years now. My family and friends have always told me that I am an amazing cook.

I have been changing family recipes into more healthier versions since I was hospitalized. I have also been testing them all out on my extended family and they REALLY love them. They especially love my Greek and Egyptian dishes that were passed down from family members. I have included many of those recipes in this book.

So, dear reader, enjoy the hard work that went into changing these recipes to help my family get healthier. These dishes are for you and your family so you too can enjoy healthy nutritious foods that are great tasting and will not spike your sugar or insulin.

I share the knowledge I have gained and the recipes I have tweaked, along with the baby steps I took to change behaviors that my doctors and I thought would NEVER change.

I am feeling better one day at a time. Weight loss and getting healthy takes work, dedication, and consistency. It isn't about quick fixes! I wish you all good health.

Happy cooking and eating,

OPA!

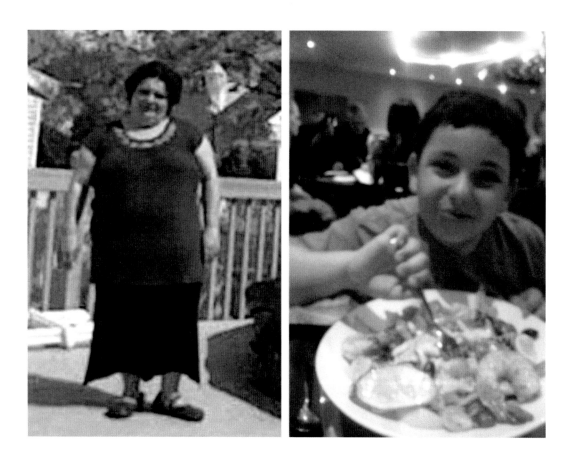

Section I

My Story

My Timeline

Healthier Day-By-Day

Forms & Action Steps

Resource Books

Resource Websites

My Story

Raised in a Greek family, most of our social gatherings are always around food. If you have ever been to a Greek restaurant you know that the foods taste amazing and we pride ourselves on our cooking. In fact, you cannot go to a Greek's house and NOT EAT!! They get very hurt!! So, that is how I ended up at 330 pounds by 42 years old.

Being brought up Greek in the 80's and 90's means you ate dishes with loads of butter, Crisco oil, salt, MSG, and white flour. The meats were high in fat content, foods were fried in toxic oil, the desserts were high in sugar, and there was a ton of bread. Well, at least, that's how I grew up!

In general, olive oil is our top ingredient in almost every dish and vegetable oil is commonly used for fried foods. The more I learned the more I switched out for myself and my family. About 3 years ago, I learned that olive oil becomes rancid when cooked on high heat. It becomes carcinogenic to our bodies, which means having the potential to grow our cancer cells. We all have those cells, keeping them from multiplying is the key to a long life.

DO WE REALLY NEED EXTRA TOXINS THESE DAYS??

In my recipes, to make them healthier for my family, I switched out olive oil for coconut oil. They didn't like the taste originally so I did it slowly ½ olive oil and ½ coconut oil for a while and suddenly they didn't notice the difference.

Recently, I learned that coconut oil is also not an oil to be used on high heat, so I switched to avocado oil. I do use olive oil in many of my recipes in this book. The difference is that I now add it at the end of the cooking process or I give you the option to slowly switch over to avocado oil for your family. Most Greek dishes tend to spike sugar levels and cause cholesterol issues.

I knew I had to do something if I wanted to change my health and the potential of my son's health. I didn't want these illnesses passed down to my son and I wanted my husband and I to live a long and healthy life. I didn't just want all of us to be healthy, I wanted us to feel healthy and look healthy FOREVER!

I started shifting out ingredients that I had learned are no longer serving our bodies and began replacing those ingredients with healthy and wholesome ingredients that I knew would benefit our immune systems and benefit my family's health. It took a few years of tweaking and testing the new recipes out on my immediate extended Greek family. I finally struck gold this past year. They all liked the tastes as well as the textures. While doing this shifting of ingredients I also brought back some recipes that I hadn't cooked in years that were passed down from my ancestors.

These foods were very healthy without any tweaking and weren't eaten very often by my extended family members anymore. I decided to cook them up and serve them at family gatherings as a way to share the love of family members who have passed. Everyone especially loved the old Greek dishes so I am sharing many of them with you in this cookbook.

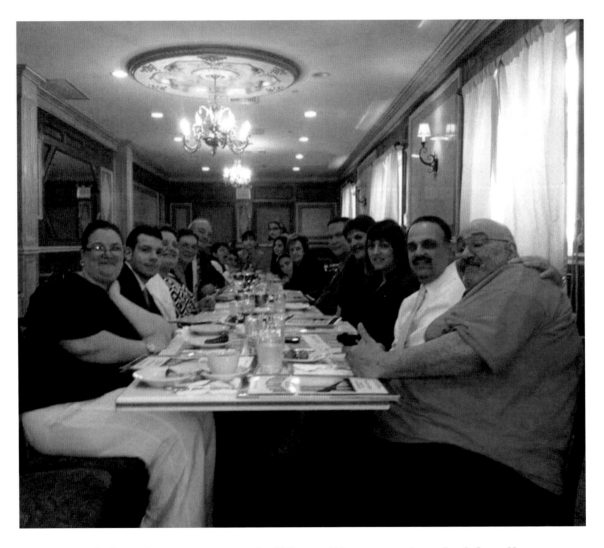

**Celebrating my mom's life, with my extended family,
rather than eating my sad feelings about losing her.
Now we get together in June every year to make new memories.**

I have dedicated this book to the most important person in my life, my mother who instilled in me the love of cooking since I was a young girl. My earliest memories were baking Greek cookies during the holidays, for my dolls. They always burned because they were too small. I dedicated this book to her because she passed away at 47 years old from many health complications. She suffered for years and now that I am getting older I realize I have the same complications.

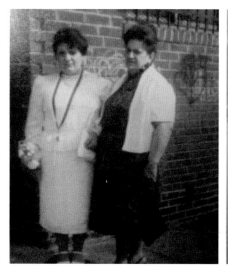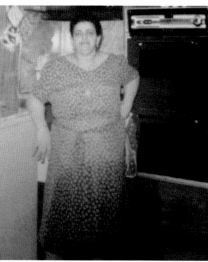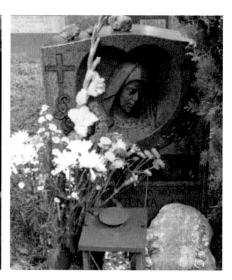

My 8ᵗʰ Grade Graduation Mom 15 Days Before Passing   My Mom's Grave

Since I was very young, my family had always wondered why I was overweight. They couldn't understand why I kept gaining weight, even when I wasn't eating poorly or that much. For years I suffered with symptoms of diabetes and I could never understand why my body wouldn't lose weight unless I restricted myself to 500 calories per day. In the picture below, I am the child in the back. My brother, Jimmy, is in front next to my mom.

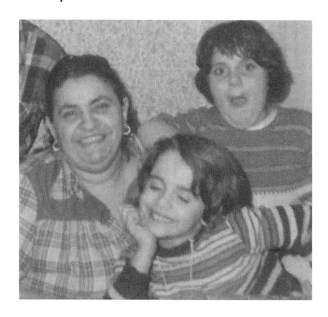

Now at 50 years old I have finally found out that all of the symptoms I have been dealing with are categorized as insulin resistance and a metabolism disorder.

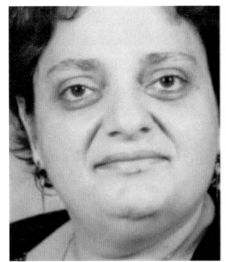 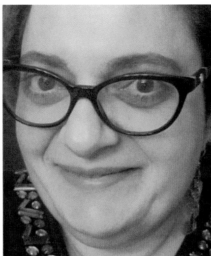 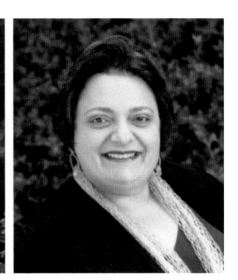

In picture on left, 2010, I looked worse than my mother did before she died at age 47. I just hit 50 and I am thrilled.

I long to support young girls in understanding themselves and their symptoms. I want them to not have to go through the torture I have put myself through for the past 50 years: Not being able to lose the weight, not being able to move freely as I would like to as a young girl, being made fun of, missed periods for months at a time, and not being able to get pregnant, having to take birth control and hormones to regulate my periods.

My journey towards better health has been bitter sweet with many ups and downs. What I have learned about myself through all of this is that when I fall down, no matter how hard, I CRY, I PROCESS, and then I always get up to face life again.

So many torturous things that weren't even needed. If I had only known the signs to look for and had put time into learning more about my metabolism disorder, I would have learned that it all stemmed from an unhealthy gut microbiome: A community of microorganisms that live in our guts and if balanced keep us healthy, when unbalanced cause dysbiosis and leave us vulnerable to illness.

One thing I do notice now as I am getting older and wiser is that I make the time to help my body heal. In the past, I looked for quick fixes! Let me tell you, if you are looking for a quick fix to getting rid of Insulin Resistance, FORGET ABOUT IT!! It doesn't exist!!

My symptoms started at 5 years old. I always had a dark ring around my neck. In fact, I remember my grandmother wanting to scrub it off when she helped me bathe. This is a picture of my neck that was taken in November of 2016.

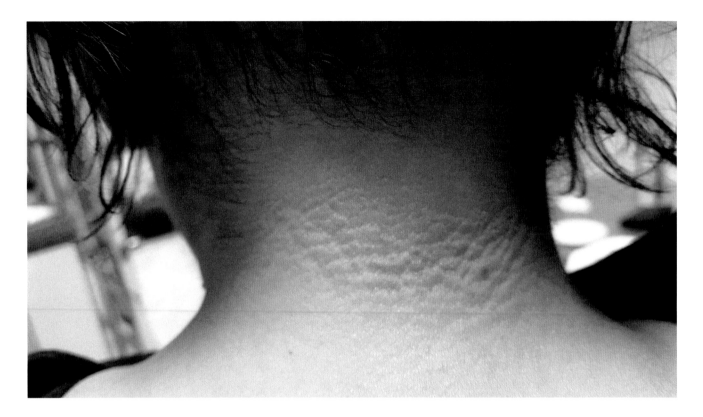

My memories from when I was 10 years old were of always being hungry, hiding food and always being scolded for eating. In my teen years and early 20's I had a big bloated belly, anxiety attacks, missed periods, Polycystic Ovary Syndrome or PCOS, panic attacks, and the worst symptom of all was that I didn't ovulate. This meant I couldn't conceive a child.

As I headed into my mid 40's the symptoms got worse, I was diagnosed with diabetes, panic attacks, and my mood changes really began to fluctuate. The worst symptoms were depression, moodiness, and brain fog.

After loads of hormones and 3 miscarriages I did finally have one beautiful son. This miracle happened only because I was ALWAYS aware that my body had some health issue and I couldn't digest simple carbs.

I always tried to avoid sugar and carbs but I didn't know what I had to do to help myself heal from these illnesses forever.

Years later after being put on numerous medications I realized that the cure had been right in front of me all along. It was my daily nutrition and my chronic stress!! It was frustrating to think about the years of trial and error, hard work, and persistence that didn't pay off until I figured out what to do.

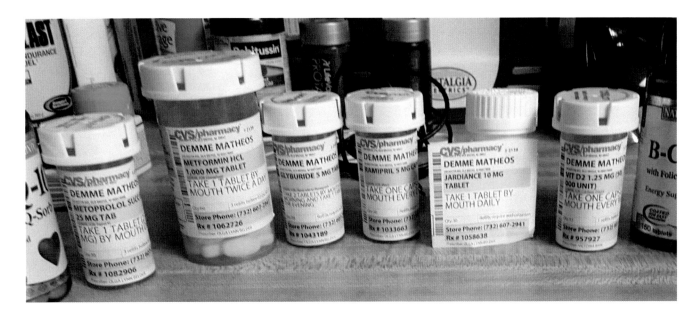

**I was on meds for Type 2 Diabetes, Pain, Anxiety, Post Traumatic Stress, Blood Pressure, Depression, COPD, High Cholesterol, 2 for heart, a total of 10. Four years later my doctors reduced me to 6 meds.
Two years after that I was down to 3 meds.**

Fast forward till today, I was told by my general doctor a few months ago that I can stop all diabetes medicines. I decided to wean myself off of them slowly this time. I have cut them down to half and I monitor my numbers closely. They are steadily stable at 100 - 120 in am. The goal is to cut them in half again by Christmas 2018 and by June 2019 I should be off of them all together.

The most important thing I have done so far, is learning to listen to my body. I now share with others, the steps I took and am still currently taking to reach my ultimate goal of health in order to feel great, look great, and not be on any medications. This is the reason for this cookbook.

My Timeline

1958: Demme's parents were married in America. Her father was born in Greece and her mother was born in US. They were both from Greek families. When Demme's father was 19 years old, he started working on cargo ships in order to help support his extended family. This allowed him many adventures around the world. Demme's mother worked at her parents dry cleaning shop in Brooklyn, NY. When she was 16 a cute sailor stepped into their shop. As they were chatting they realized that they were from the same Greek island. Her parents were delighted and they were married 3 years later in 1958.

1963: Demme's sister Annie was born

1968: Demme was born (Demme's sister was 5)

1970: Demme's little brother Jimmy was born (Demme was 2 years old)

June 1, 1985: Mom's Death (Demme, Age 15½)

June 1986: Demme graduated from high school. Her widowed father went to Greece to get re-married. His family had arranged a marriage for him so he left America to meet his bride-to-be.

August 1986: Demme went to Greece to join her father. This was 1 year after her mother's passing. Demme fell in love with Greece and asked her father if she could stay there. He said, "I can't leave you here alone. What if we get you engaged." Her family found some prospective suitors. Demme picked one of them, one she felt she could get along with temporarily. She figured she'd stay engaged for a little while and break off the engagement. Right after they were engaged her father told her she had to marry this man. He was 4 years older than Demme. This ended up being an arranged marriage. Demme's dad got re-married August, 1986.

January 1987: Demme's arranged marriage took place.

April 1987: Demme's step-brother Peter was born in America and Demme was married and living in Greece.

Summer of 1987: Demme visited America and saw Peter for the first time. He was 6 months old. She loves her step-brother. They have always been very close. Neither one of them use the word 'step'. They consider themselves brother and sister.

Demme stayed in America with her husband for about a year. Her husband didn't like America and wanted to go back to Greece.

March 1988: Demme and her husband moved back to Greece.

March 22, 1993: Demme's father had his first stroke (Demme Age 25). Within days Demme and her husband arrived in America.

June 1993: Demme's husband had an argument with her father and Demme had a huge argument with her husband. She was fed up with the domestic abuse and sent him packing.

Christmas 1993: Demme went to Greece to take care of the things she had left in Greece. Her husband began begging her to stay. In January of '94 she attempted to leave and her extended family members, living there in Greece, physically stopped her from leaving. She set plans into motion to sneak away the following month and she accomplished that goal. She fled Greece and moved back to America in February 1994.

August 1994: Demme returned to Greece to sign her divorce papers and make everything legal and final.

September 1995: Demme met her current husband, Essam Eliraky in America. They were destined to meet. He is the love of her life and her best friend.

April 1996: Her dad passed away from a massive stroke, 3 years exactly from the date he had first one. Demme was inspired to become a Speech Pathologist while helping her father get back his speech after his first stroke. She continued this work for 15 years in various settings.

2003: Demme and Essam were married. She experienced 3 Miscarriages: One before their son was born and two after their only child. Adam, Demme and Essam's son was born in 2004.

May 2010: Demme thought she was having a heart-attack. She was hospitalized for Angina, High Blood Pressure, Anxiety, High Cholesterol, and Chronic Obstructive Pulmonary Disease or COPD a lung disease.

June 2010 Started Weight Watchers: Lost 60 pounds by 2012.

April 2011: Demme walked her first 5K race despite issues with her legs.

December 2011: Took a family trip to Eygpt to see Essam's family. Demme was able to do more activities than before her hospitalization. She hadn't even realized she hadn't really been living her life.

April 2012: Signed up to walk a 5K race with her son. Demme wasn't able to finish due to leg pain. Adam finished the race running with 3 trainers even though he wanted to give up. He was so excited to have finished the race.

May 2012: Her first grade teacher, Ms. Boutross, saw her online teaching people how to shift their health and told her to sign-up for the IIN Health Coach Certification. Demme listened and completed her certification in 2013.

June 2012: Demme signed up to participate in a Mini-Triathlons at the gym: Biked 6 miles on the exercise bike, walked 2 miles on the treadmill, and swam 15 laps in the pool.

September 2012: She was doing really well, 70 pounds down since her hospitalization. Then her sister had a stroke. Demme 'forgot that Demme existed' while constantly traveling, 6 hours round trip, to and from the hospital, while not eating or drinking much. She would grab something from the hospital cafeteria and eat while she was driving home.

October 2012: Hurricane Sandy hit New Jersey (no heat, no electric, no running water for 7 days). No gas available at the gas station so Demme couldn't visit her sister and was also unable to make contact with her.

November 2012: Essam was in a car accident and consequently lost his job. He went into full on depression for 4 years. About the same time, Demme's sister was moved to a long term physical rehab center. Most of the patients there were elderly and Annie hated it there. Demme was fighting with the doctors and staff every single day advocating for her sister and ended up getting Annie a private room.

February 2013: "Fuck this you are going back to the gym," she told herself. Her son was 8 years old and being bullied at school for his weight. He was starting to have hormone issues as well. The kids were teasing him about his 'man boobs,' which were signs of a hormone imbalance because of age and weight.

Severe financial stress: Going to the gym helped Demme move past the financial stress. A few months later she was eating healthier and becoming a priority once again.

April 2013: In January Demme signed up to RUN in a 5K race in April. She hired a trainer and hurt her left knee during training, although she was able to walk the event.

May 2014: She had knee Replacement Surgery, the had a long recovery with lots of pain. Demme found out that her whole body had been compensating for years which added more difficulties and discomfort to the healing process. Demme started Aqua Classes to aide in her recovery.

November 2014: Essam had neck surgery, a fusion. Demme hurt her back helping him. His depression got worse from all of the recovery pain.

2015 New Year's Resolution: To stop focusing on weight loss and start focusing on self-care. AKA one massage a month. This was the beginning of Demme's 'Taking Care of Me Campaign' and to remind her that she is the priority. Demme got off of sleeping pills, as well as her meds for anxiety, blood pressure, and COPD meds.

May 2015: Essam had spinal surgery and his depression worsened.

October 2015: Demme hired a bodybuilder/nutritionist. She didn't really lose weight, lost fat and inches. In total Demme only lost 6 pounds of fat and gained 22 pounds of muscle. She was pissed and yet felt strong. Still getting sick often and being put on antibiotics. Started eating more micronutrients.

April 2016: Found Dr. George Kosmides on Periscope. Demme was delighted to find and eventually meet a doctor who talked about the health things she had gotten figured out. She stopped eating fruits after 5pm and lost 15 pounds. Her doctor took her off of all her meds except her prescriptions for diabetes.

May 2016: Essam had a heart attack for his birthday. Lovely!

October 2016: Demme's doctor reduced her diabetes medications. She was hospitalized for kidney stones from her blood sugar levels going up and down like crazy! This also resulted in chronic yeast infections. Demme had to see a urologist and a pneumologist every 2 to 3 months to make sure she was no longer developing kidney stones or headed for kidney disease.

2017 New Year's Resolution: Taking care of 'myself' even more. New goal of 2 massages per month. Kept working on getting her immune system healthier. Became more responsible on her choices for cheating. Hired a personal trainer to keep her accountable for going to the gym through the winter months, which was harder for her when it came to consistency.

December 2016: Went to Chichen Itza, Mexico with her husband and son. Walked the whole time. Felt like she could heal herself fully.

2017 Last Cardiologist Appointment: Demme had dropped 25 pounds. This was the doctor that a year ago had said, "Just shut your mouth and stop eating." Now he was saying, "Keep doing what you are doing, because you are doing amazing and I don't need to see you anymore. He also took her off her blood pressure meds."

July 2017: Traveled throughout Greece and Egypt with her immediate family, visiting relatives in both countries. Before the trip Demme worried that such an active and lengthy trip might be a problem for her. She ended up doing really well and kept up with everyone. They hiked, toured museums, and monasteries hidden in caves. They walked all the way up to the Acropolis. She had some issues and yet she got there. Demme made amends with some family members after her mindfulness assessment adjustments. After the trip, Demme held steady on all of her commitments.

November 2017: Demme and her family took a trip to Arizona for her birthday. It was a Soul adventure where she was able to go deep in order to help herself discover how she could become more mindful on a daily basis and stay in her body.

2018 New Year's Resolution: Hungry, Eat. Not Hungry, STOP! Mindfulness and do not listen to other people's protocols. Listen to 'my' body instead. This felt like it would be a perfect year. Then boom!

January 2018—Life's 'Friggin' Curve Balls: Dr. George Kosmides passed away. Demme lost momentum. His Zoom group voted Demme in as one of the leaders, in order to keep the group running. After about 2 months she told the group she just couldn't do anymore classes for them. He had over 500 followers in that group and she was sad to let it go. She had just enrolled in a 6 month Gut Health certification course through IIN. It was all a bit much at the time.

March 2018: Demme tried some new things she was learning from her gut health course and they made a huge difference. She ended up trying too many things at one time so she wasn't sure which ones were working. She decided to keep going.

April 2018: She hired a doctor of functional medicine and found out that she had a parasite. Demme was advised to get off all of her supplements and start this particular doctors protocol. Things went crazy from there!

May 2018: Demme signed up for a book course through IIN, met Irina B. Stuchinsky an IIN grad who had just published her book through Linda Vettrus-Nichols and had shared that information with Demme.

August 2018: Demme went on an Alaskan cruise with her husband and her son. She worried about her bad knee, the one that could use surgery for a knee replacement, she is holding off until January of 2019. Everything went well in Alaska, even with tons of walking. This trip really brought her inward. She was overwhelmed with the beauty of the wildlife. It was a spiritual time with a sense of a deep calling. She would indeed write her first book.

November 2018: Demme published, this, her first book/cookbook, wasn't sick all year, so no anti-biotics or even pain meds.

Healthier Day-By-Day

A few times in my journey I tried to be perfect! Perfection doesn't exist! DON'T BEAT YOURSELF UP!!! Accept what happened, learn the lesson, and move forward.

No one diet or lifestyle works for everyone. Each person's nutritional needs are individual and based on a number of varying factors such as lifestyle, occupation, climate, age, gender, culture, and religion. Lifestyle needs are individual as well; what works for one person may not work for another with regard to relationships, exercise, career, spirituality, and physical activity.

Additionally, our bodies change over time so it's important to check-in with yourself and your body every so often and note what needs attention.

Take a Picture for Your Records: It's always great to have a before and after picture just to see where you started. Your skin may change, your nails may get stronger. Sometimes the changes are subtle, you will definitely see differences. Take measurements of your body. Go see your doctor and get blood work done before starting changes in your diet. In other words, get a baseline read.

Know Your Why: What drives you?

Note What You Consume Daily: Without changing anything write down what you consume daily for one week. Awareness of what is currently going on is huge!

Drink More Water: Half of your body weight in water. Our bodies need water to function correctly. One thing that stuck in my head from school was that our organs need water to function properly. Heart attacks are connected to water absorption and pituitary. So drink up!

Add More Leafy Green Veggies to Your Diet: Yeah, I know, blah-blah-blah!! I will be showing you, throughout my cookbook series, how to make them tasty.

Avoid Drinking Sugary Drinks: Reduce your intake of them as you start and slowly you will not want them anymore.

Start Walking or Going to the Gym for 30 Minutes Daily: Did you know that this step will lower your cholesterol? It will also: Raise your good cholesterol, lower your blood pressure, strengthen your heart, strengthen your lungs, improve your circulation issues, assist in ridding your body of excess water weight, help you stay younger, reduce anxiety, etc. The list goes on and on as far as all of the benefits you get when you do this.

Do Something Just For 'YOU' EVERY DAY for 60 Minutes: Go for a massage, listen to an audiobook, go have coffee with a friend, go bowling, etc.

Sit and Breathe for 5 Minutes: There is a breathing exercise I use that is great for assisting the Vegas nerve, which is responsible for many bodily functions. This is done by alternating breathing in through one nostril and letting that breath out through the other nostril. Simply press your index finger on the side of your nose. When breathing in, hold the breath for 4 counts. Use the other nostril and breathe out for 4 counts.

Journal: Keep a journal of when you do go off track, not only with food but with anything you had planned. What takes you off your goals? Where does it happen? Who is around?

Have Fun: Start making more time to have fun. *(ex. go bowling, go to the movies, paint a pot, paint and wine, play pool, join a gym with a friend, go for a walk with a friend in the mall, etc.)*

Choose One Focus: Pick one thing that you can do daily and do it consistently.(ex. Drink more water than yesterday, walk for 10 minutes, etc.)

Consistent Focus: Stay consistent with your 'one thing' and once you get that down, as a lifestyle habit, add one more thing that you can do. Remember, it is a process to get healthy. It doesn't happen overnight.

Go Easy on Yourself: Avoid punishing yourself for not doing everything perfect.

Avoid Comparisons: Everyone is in a different place on their health and life journey so don't compare yourself to ANYONE else!

It's a Journey, Not a Quick Fix: The journey will have dips and sometimes you will not feel well and other times you will see great improvements. Give your body a chance to heal from the inside out. It didn't take you a few weeks or months to get unhealthy. Becoming healthier won't happen right away.

Signs of a Healthier You: You may see signs of thicker and stronger nails, better looking skin, improved sleep, lowered diabetes numbers, more energy, lower blood pressure, better sight, or lower cholesterol before you see the scale move. Your body is healing your organs first then the outside.

List Your Health Issues: Make a list of all your health issues now so you can see the improvements as you heal your body.

Bedtime Guideline for Eating Fruit: Avoid eating fruit 3 hours before bed. This spikes your sugar levels.

Eat More Protein: Try to support your body each day by making sure you eat some protein. Did you ever notice that as people age they lose their leg muscle mass? It's because they are not supporting their bodies with enough protein to sustain their muscles. Protein is needed by all of our organs first and foremost. If the body is not supported it will take it from the leg and buttocks muscles first.

Stay Clear of White Foods: White flour, white pasta, sugar, white or whole wheat bread. Limit or avoid these foods because they are known to cause inflammation in the gut. This causes issues with proper digestion. Everyone reacts differently.

Avoid Negative People: Stay away from negative people and situations. This is very important. Some people are energy vampires. Even Picasso was known to be an energy vampire.

Limit Coffee & All Caffeine: Studies show that caffeine triggers inflammation of the gut lining and causes digestion to slow down.

Limit Processed Foods: These foods are made in a laboratory. They can not be easily broken down and properly digested. This can cause holes in the lining of the intestinal walls. This creates mucus because the body rushes to heal these holes. Allergies and food sensitivities many times originate with what is called leaky gut.

Read Labels & Look at Ingredients: Be very alert to what is written on food labels. If sugar is the first ingredient, the product is mostly sugar. There are many forms of sugar. Be a detective.

Avoid Overcooking Veggies: This takes all of the nutrients out.

Add Lemon to Your Water: Assists liver in in flushing out unwanted toxins.

Create New Habits: Once you have eliminated what does not serve you, you can begin adding 'one new healthy habit' to your lifestyle, after you become consistent with your new habit.

Avoid What 'Stresses' You Out: Do what is easy on your body. LISTEN TO YOUR BODY. Why? Because it's the boss and it knows best!!

Be Honest with Yourself: Are you really hungry? Are you thirsty? Are you bored? or Are you feeling alone? LISTEN CLOSELY!!!

Quick Fix Diets: All you are doing is losing water weight with those quick fix diets. No real changes will happen in your health without changing your habits slowly step-by-step.

Everyone is different and each client has different circumstances and health issues. What works for one person may not work for someone else.

My typical clients tend to not like vegetables or exercising. They feel like they have tried everything to lose weight, get off of meds, and/or just get healthy in general.

I REMIND THEM THAT...

IT'S NOT ABOUT DIETING, ITS ABOUT CREATING A HEALTHY LIFESTYLE, CHANGE THAT LASTS FOREVER!!!

Forms & Action Steps

Self-Assessment

Your Why

Short Term Goals

What is Your Story?

Long Term Goals

Journal

Letter to My Future Self

Bucket List

Decluttering

Self-Assessment

What was going on in other parts of my life made a huge difference on my food choices. Who 'friggin' knew that if I wasn't feeling fulfilled in ALL areas of my life, that it would make a difference when it came to my food choices?

Once I started my health journey, I'd choose broccoli and a lean protein. I wasn't even aware that when I was stressed, for example, about my finances, I would automatically chose a burger and fries or four slices of pizza. I was surprised how much being out of balance in various areas of my life effected my food choices.

It is important to understand what is important to us, what we take comfort from, and to what extent it plays out in ALL areas of our lives. The Self-Assessment form on the following page keeps me mindful of where I am at any given time in my life.

Filling out this chart is a fabulous way to track yourself and your life goals whatever they might be.

Feel free to make several copies of it for yourself. Make sure to fill out the assessment when you start your journey. I like to fill it out monthly or when I feel I have slipped in some areas.

Guilt

When I started looking at the various areas of my life, I would take my mindfulness assessment, and chose one particular area to focus on. The problem was that the area I chose to focus on would improve and other areas tended to suffer. For example, when I focused on getting to the gym, my nutrition would suffer. Instead of feeling guilty, I decided to not focus on just one thing.

The most interesting thing that happened was that I began to put my needs before others. I used to forget I existed when something crazy happened in my life. I wasn't even on the list. It was extra important for me to make myself a priority.

In my upbringing, it was considered selfish to think about myself first. This lesson kept coming up for me until I finally realized that this was to be my main focus in ALL areas of my life. Keep myself first and remind myself that I am number one.

My health is not just important to me. It's important to everyone around me. My family and friends depend on me to be healthy! Moving through life with this framework in mind is very freeing and a great way to make sure that guilt isn't part of the problem.

Each step forward brought about a new awareness. I learned what triggered me and what I needed to do the next time I encountered that person, food, or situation. Including what had spiked my sugar and what had made me feel better and healthier.

Digging deeper with those probing questions, I finally figured out that exercise was a motivator for me. It didn't matter what type of exercise I did, I just needed to get out for about 30 minutes every day.

Perfection

A few times in my journey I tried to be perfect and guess what I discovered? Perfection doesn't exist! Sooooooo, NO NEED TO BEAT YOURSELF UP!!! Accept your slip ups. Accept what happened, figure it out and apply the lesson learned, then move forward.

Slip Ups

Too many times when we slip up we go into this mindset and begin to give ourselves permission to continue for another day, then week, then month, you get the picture. We've all been there!

The problem with slip ups is that we end up ruining all of our hard work. I remember one time eating a chocolate chip muffin. I was so upset, I began to cry. Then I realized that it was a damn muffin! That muffin didn't make me gain all my weight. It took years and many muffins, not to mention neglecting the other areas of my life to get me where I was so slip ups can bring us into perspective or we can allow them to trigger us.

In order to avoid slip ups and the ensuing guilt trip, think about your Why!

Forgiveness

For me, doing a mindful self-assessment creates a huge relief from the guilt and slip ups in my life. It also reminds me that the unhealthy life I once led wasn't my fault. Many factors, that were not in my control at the time, brought me to an unhealthy state.

However, I can change my destiny now that I know better.

Do the best you can until you know better.

Then when you know better, do better.

-Maya Angelou

Remember: Eating healthy IS a LIFESTYLE *forever*, NOT A FUCKING DIET!!!!

Self-Assessment
My Mindfulness Chart (MMC)

Date: _____/_____/_____

Joy or Happiness	1	2	3	4	5	6	7	8	9	10
Physical Activity or Movement	1	2	3	4	5	6	7	8	9	10
Mental Health	1	2	3	4	5	6	7	8	9	10
Spiritual Health	1	2	3	4	5	6	7	8	9	10
Overall Health	1	2	3	4	5	6	7	8	9	10
Meditation	1	2	3	4	5	6	7	8	9	10
Relationships: Family & Friends	1	2	3	4	5	6	7	8	9	10
Food Sensitivities	1	2	3	4	5	6	7	8	9	10
Allergies	1	2	3	4	5	6	7	8	9	10
Triggers	1	2	3	4	5	6	7	8	9	10
Anxiety and/or Stress	1	2	3	4	5	6	7	8	9	10
Libido	1	2	3	4	5	6	7	8	9	10
Sleep	1	2	3	4	5	6	7	8	9	10
Eat and Drink Consistently	1	2	3	4	5	6	7	8	9	10
Creativity & Fun	1	2	3	4	5	6	7	8	9	10
Financial Satisfaction	1	2	3	4	5	6	7	8	9	10
Career Satisfaction	1	2	3	4	5	6	7	8	9	10
Continuing Education	1	2	3	4	5	6	7	8	9	10
Cooking for Self and Family	1	2	3	4	5	6	7	8	9	10
Healthy Living Environment	1	2	3	4	5	6	7	8	9	10

Make A few Copies of this chart

Directions: Fill out the date. Assess where you are at on a scale of 1 to 10: Ten being the most satisfied/fulfilled. Circle the number that best reflects where you feel you are in your life at this moment in time.

Be Creative: Use this chart to get an initial baseline. Then use it when you want to assess where you are from time to time. For example: Monthly or when you feel you have slipped in some areas or you want to see where you need support.

Your Why

What is Your Why?

I started my health journey by taking a look at my WHY. My wake up call was my trip to the Emergency Room. It took me hours to decide to go and then I thought about my son. Once I started realizing I could die, I knew that I didn't want to leave my son motherless.

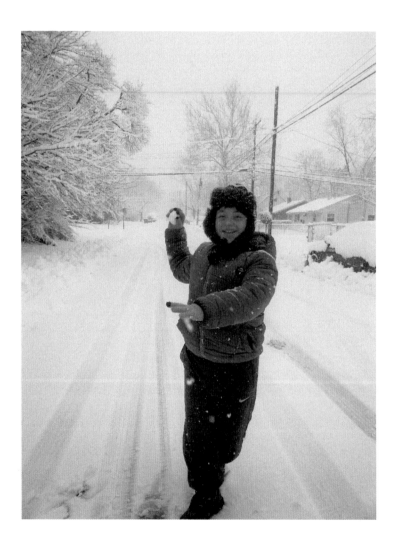

My Why!

What is your why?

Answering this question is your next step. Once you know your Why ask yourself, "Why is this my why?" For example, if your goal is to lose weight ask yourself, "Why?" My goal was to not die. My why was my son. I didn't want to leave him motherless. It broke my heart to think of him being all alone, even though he would have had his father. My mother died when I was 15, I felt all alone after she died.

Once You Know Your Why

If your 'why' is to lose weight then ask yourself, "Why do I want to lose this weight?" If it's about getting healthier ask yourself, "Why do I want to get healthier?"

If you would like to decrease or get off of your meds all together ask yourself, "Why do I want to get off my meds?"

My 'why' was my son. Staying alive and being healthier for my son was and is my main goal.

I also thought back to when I was younger. How much I hated seeing my mom sit on the side lines. How I hated seeing my mom sick. I hated seeing my mom take more than 15 medicines and having to prick her finger daily. I watched her give herself insulin shots every morning and I said to myself, "That will never be me!"

I remember the day we lost my mom and how it felt and now the feeling of missing my mom daily and how it feels that she is not here with me to see me and her grandchildren. So that experience reinforced my 'why.'

If that wasn't a motivation I don't know what could drive me even more.

Well, I guess the other thing that was my driving force was that I never ever thought I would be the sedentary person on the side lines. Holding the jackets, and cameras while everyone else was living life to its fullest!!!

Reality is, that's exactly what happened! I had slowly become my mother!

That is when I finally decided FUCK THIS!! I WILL GET HEALTHY IF IT IS THE LAST THING I 'FRIGGIN' DO!! I began to become the role model for my son and many friends and family who followed me.

Each step forward I learned something new about myself: What triggered my bad eating? What I needed to stay away from? Who triggered me and what I needed to do the next time I encountered that person? What spiked my sugar and what made me feel better and healthier?

Digging deeper with those probing questions, I finally figured out that exercise was a motivator for me. It didn't matter what type of exercise, I just needed to get out for about 30 minutes every day.

I have included a worksheet for you to figure out your Why. Follow the directions and be honest with yourself. Make sure your Why is motivating enough for you to reach your goals.

Throughout my health journey there have been certain things that have gotten in my way. Some were under my control and others were not. For example, when my husband was dealing with depression after his accident I chose to not let that get in my way and I headed back to the gym.

My 'Why?' Worksheet

Why do you want to reach this goal? *For example, "I want to be able to play with my children."* Journal reasons and make sure you dig deep and state what is holding you back right now from reaching this goal.

_____

_____

_____

_____

_____

_____

_____

_____

_____

_____

_____

_____

_____

_____

_____

_____

Date ___/___/_____

Short Term Goals

As you know, everything in my life came to a screeching halt 8 years ago when I was admitted to the hospital on Mother's Day. I felt like I was having a heart attack and my immune system was very weak.

My then 6-year-year old son cried every night, thinking I was going to die! I promised myself, those 12 long days before I was discharged, that I would get serious about my health. As you know, I was diagnosed with various illnesses and one of them was Type 2 Diabetes.

It was very scary!

I remembered hearing a woman talking about how she had started her journey towards better health. Like me, she couldn't go for a walk.

Her advice was great! She started walking from her house to her mailbox and back, once a day. I said to myself, "YOU CAN DO THAT!" So I set my goal for 5 minutes, walked until my timer went off, and then walked back home. Five minutes turned miraculously into 10 minutes of walking. So that was my first goal. AND WHERE IT ALL BEGAN!!

One Month Goals

A goal must be do-able. Choose something that you can actually do. Add more water to your day. Make sure you are getting outside to walk, even if it's a goal to park further away from your destination.

My One Month Goal Worksheet

One month from today I promise to myself that I will...

_____

_____

_____

I will reach this goal by taking the following steps...

1._____

2._____

3._____

I will stay accountable to myself and stay consistent, because this is going to help me achieve a better me in 'all' ways.

Signature _____

Date___/___/___

No excuses!!

Live as a healthier you each day!

What is Your Story?

We all have a story that we share when we meet new people. It sounds like a broken record. It plays over and over and we start to believe it and begin to live it. So what is your story? Be honest with yourself. No one else has to see this. Once you begin to be honest with yourself, things will automatically shift for you and become more positive. Xoxoox

_____

_____

_____

_____

_____

_____

_____

_____

_____

_____

_____

Six months from today I promise myself that I will...

_____

_____

_____

I will reach this goal by taking the following steps...

1._____

2._____

3._____

I will stay accountable to myself and stay consistent, because this is going to help me achieve a better me in all ways.

Signature _____

Date____/____/_____

No excuses!!

Better healthier you each day!

I'm Accountable To Me!

What can I do to move myself forward toward my goals this week?

Drink more water_____

Eat more veggies_____

I am listening to my body and what it is telling me about...

Sleep? _____

Rest?_____

Fun?_____

Exercise?_____

Family time?_____

Friends?_____

Cooking at home?_____

Finances?_____

Spirituality?_____

Stress? _____

Positive?_____

Consistent?_____

What can I tweak this week to help me be more accountable to my goals?

_____

_____

_____

_____

_____

Long Term Goals

The deeper I got into nutrition and mindset the more I worked on my health and the healthier I got. I remember finally realizing that I needed to step back and out of certain situations.

It was crazy at first because I couldn't believe that I actually was saying NO to various situations proposed to me.

I finally saw that I was stagnant in my life, not only in my weight. I had held onto my mom's things for years. I had held onto so much stuff. I needed to declutter my body, my home, and my mind. THAT WAS A VERY HARD SHIFT INDEED and IF I was able to DO IT, EVERYONE CAN!!! I finally had realized that instead of doing what needed to be done in my own home and life, I was always avoiding it by helping others and trying to escape my reality by going out for coffee or doing whatever was going on in other people's lives.

I WASN'T LIVING MY LIFE TO ITS FULLEST!! That's when I decided to push forward. I hired a *De-clutter-er*. Wow, was she ever AMAZING!! She definitely had a completely different mindset than I did.

The more I let go of STUFF! The better I felt!

I donated, sold, and let go of so many things. As I let go of 'stuff' new and wonderful things would come into my life. I began to work hard on the decluttering of things as well as on decluttering my mind.

Things became clearer each time I went deeper. Yes it was rough and yet it had the benefit of a detox each time.

Journal

Journal Daily or Weekly

Worst thing that has ever happened to me in my whole life so far:

_____

_____

_____

_____

_____

_____

_____

_____

_____

_____

_____

Letter to My Future Self

(Write this letter and put it in an envelope, send it to a close relative or friend with a self-addressed envelope and ask them to send it back to you in 2 years from the date you sent it.)

Date _____

Dear _____,

Signed with lots of love,

Bucket List

Things I want to do and places I want to visit:

1.

2.

3.

4.

5.

6.

7.

8.

9.

10.

11.

12.

13.

14.

15.

16.

Decluttering
(People & Things Lists)

Things or people holding me from reaching my goals....

_____

_____

_____

_____

_____

_____

Actions I will take to overcome these setbacks...

_____

_____

_____

_____

Resource Books

LIFE without DIABETES, by Dr. George Kosmides, DC, CCN

The Big Leap, by Gay Hendricks

The Seven Spiritual Laws of Success, by Deepak Chopra

*Loving What Is, b*y Byron Katie

The Work, by Byron Katie

The Habits of Happy People, by Thomas J. Slominski, MA

YOU Are a BADASS: HOW TO STOP DOUBTING YOUR GREATNESS AND START LIVING AN AWESOME LIFE, by Jen Sincero

*The Motivation Manifesto 9 Declarations to Claim Your Personal Power, b*y Brendon Burchard

Acid & Alkaline, by Herman Aihara

Your Bodies Many Cries for Water, by Dr. Batmanghelidj, M.D

Prescription for Nutritional Healing: A Practical A-to-Z Reference to Drug-Free Remedies Using Vitamins, Minerals, Herbs & Food Supplements, Fifth Edition, by Phyllis A. Balch, C.N.C.

Resource Websites

Here is a list of websites that will give you additional resources...

www.RebootYourselfNow.com

www.DocWendel.com

www.DrBerg.com

www.PureFitWomen.fit

www.5LoveLanguages.com

www.TheWork.com (resources from Byron Katie, author of *The Work*)

www.Napo.net (find a certified declutter expert here)

www.SedonaSoulAdventures.com

www.MarsVenus.com

www.Tinkyada.com (brown rice company I use)

www.EvolutionaryHealer.com

www.LindaVettrus-Nichols.com

Section II

Appetizer & Sides Recipes

Salad & Soup Recipes

Entrée Recipes

Dessert Recipes

Drink Recipes

Appetizer & Sides Recipes

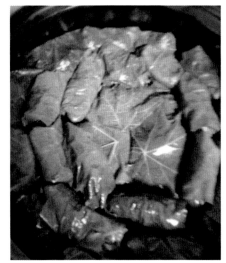 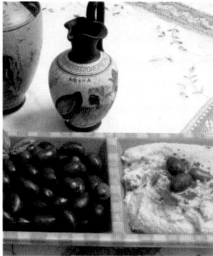 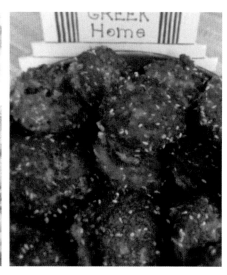

Demme's Spinach Pie

Bahia's Falafel

Kolokithokeftedes
(Zucchini Meatballs)

Tzatziki

Hummus

Gigantes Ala Eugenia

Demme's Healthier Dolmades
(Grape Leaves)

Recipes

Demme's Spinach Pie

3 pounds of fresh spinach or frozen equivalent

3 medium onions chopped

1 cup of scallions chopped

4 cloves of garlic chopped

½ cup of organic butter or avocado oil

2 cups of fresh chopped dill

Salt and pepper to taste

2-3 eggs

1 pound phyllo pastry

Melted butter as needed for phyllo

½ pound of feta cheese crumbled

8 oz ricotta cheese

Wash spinach well and cut into small pieces. Sauté the onion and garlic with ¼ of the butter until it is light golden brown. Add scallions and continue to stir until the scallions wilt just a little. Then add the spinach. Stir until everything takes on a light color. Then stir in the dill, salt, and pepper (go lightly on salt because feta already has plenty of salt). Let everything cook until water is absorbed. Pull off stove and let cool. If there is any water in mixture, drain in a colander. In another bowl beat eggs and add all cheeses, add to cooked spinach mixture and mix well.

Get a pan that is at least 2 inches deep, brush with melted butter. Lay one phyllo sheet flat on the bottom of the pan, then brush it with butter. The phyllo dough does not need to be evenly or completely buttered. Repeat this step until 8 sheets are layered in the pan. Pour the spinach and cheese mixture evenly over the phyllo. Fold the parts of the phyllo, that extend out of the pan, back over the spinach filling. It should look like an envelope or an enclosure. Brush the phyllo ends with butter and then lay down another 6-8 phyllo layers, buttering each layer. Pour remaining butter on top of the last layer, then score into square serving pieces. Bake for 30-45 minutes in a preheated oven, at 300° F. Check the bottom crust of the spinach pie by lifting slightly; look for a golden brown color before taking it out of the oven. Let stand for 30 minutes before serving.

Note: I am currently working on finding a phyllo dough that is healthier. Keep a lookout for it on my Website. www.RebootYourselfNow.com

Bahia's Falafel

This recipe will make enough to fill four, quart bags to put away in the freezer.

1 bag of fava beans

2 eggs

3 tablespoons of sesame seeds

1 tablespoon of cracked red pepper flakes

Salt and pepper

Fry in avocado oil

1 tsp baking powder

1 whole bunch of chopped fresh parsley

2 whole large chopped onions

5 cloves chopped garlic

1 whole green pepper chopped

Oil for Frying: I use avocado oil because it's one of the oils that will not go rancid when cooked on high heat. I also have tried to bake the falafels on parchment paper, but they don't come out as good and are a bit dry.

Process: Soak fava beans overnight. Rinse well. Blend in a food processor. Add onions, garlic, green pepper, parsley, and all remaining ingredients except sesame seeds. When everything is blended, place mixture in a separate bowl and mix in the sesame seeds. Separate into baggies for the freezer.

To Cook Some Now: Set some aside and add another egg into the mixture.

Add 1 tsp of baking powder to the mixture, to be used currently. Start heating a pan and add the cooking oil. As soon as the oil is ready, shape up a smooth falafel ball and flatten it into a patty. Put it into the cooking oil. Wait a bit for browning to show on edges and turn over to cook the other side. Prepare a plate with paper towels, place the cooked falafel patty on it to drain off the excess oil. Serve either in a sandwich or with a salad or just dip it in tahini. Enjoy!!

Note: *You will have approximately 48 falafels to put into the freezer. Make sure to defrost them first, bring to room temperature before cooking. Follow the same steps above for cooking the remaining falafel patties.*

Kolokithokeftedes—Zucchini Meatballs

2 pounds of small green squash grated

1 tablespoon of butter

1 cup of grated onion

1 cup of grated Kefalograviera Cheese or Pecorino Romano

1 cup of gluten free breadcrumbs

2 tablespoons of chopped fresh parsley

1 teaspoon of fresh minced mint or dried mint

2 eggs

Salt and pepper to taste (go easy on the salt, cheese already plenty of salt)

Fry in avocado oil

Clean and wash the squash. Grate squash and onion, then let stand in a colander to drain excess water out. Press down and squeeze in order to get out as much liquid as you can. Place all ingredients in a bowl. If the mixture is too soft, add more bread crumbs. Roll into balls, then flatten into patties. Fry until golden brown on each side. Let stand for 15 minutes and serve with a salad or as a side dish.

Tzatziki

1 large cucumber grated

2-3 cups of Fage Total 5% (Greek yogurt) If you can't find it, get a strained yogurt

3-4 cloves of garlic minced, depending how spicy you like it! I use more!

Salt and pepper to taste

1-2 tablespoons of Bragg Apple Cider Vinegar

2 tablespoons top grade olive oil

Clean the cucumber. Grate the cucumber; make sure to place a clean white towel under the grater to absorb the excess water. In another bowl add the yogurt, garlic, vinegar, salt, pepper, and olive oil. Mix well. Then add the grated cucumber to the mix. Stir and put in the refrigerator for 1 to 2 hours. Serve with meat, chicken or veggies. Great as a dip for veggies and chips or as a side for lamb, beef and chicken.

Hummus

1-2 cans of organic BPA free chickpeas

½ cup organic olive oil

1-2 Lemons squeezed

Salt and pepper to taste

4-5 Garlic cloves

1 tablespoon Bragg Apple Cider Vinegar

2 tablespoons of tahini paste

½ teaspoon of cumin

Red cracked pepper to taste (optional)

Black olives to garnish

Drain and rinse the canned chickpeas well. Put chickpeas into a food processor or a blender. Add lemon, garlic, olive oil, vinegar, and cumin. Blend well. Add the tahini paste, salt, and pepper to taste. Blend a bit more. You may want to do a taste test to see if you would like it spicier or saltier. At this time you could add something you feel is missing, such as more salt or pepper. Remember, you can always add more salt you cannot take it out. I love spicy foods! I also add the red cracked pepper to taste at this time. Put hummus in a glass bowl, spread nicely and evenly on top. Sprinkle a little paprika and a little olive oil on top of the hummus. Place in fridge for 1-2 hours. The longer it is in the fridge the better the taste! Serve with chips or fresh cut veggies as a dip. Goes well with falafel or zucchini balls. A great side dish too. Enjoy!!

Gigantes Ala Eugenia

1 pound of gigantes (giant white beans) dry or 1 large can gigantes

½ cup olive oil

3 large carrots chopped

2 medium onions chopped

2-3 garlic cloves chopped

2 large fresh tomatoes chopped

2-3 stalks of celery chopped

4-5 Basil leaves chopped

Note: This step is for dry beans only. If using canned beans skip this step, however make sure to rinse them first.

Soak dry beans overnight in a glass bowl. In the morning, rinse and put them in a pot of water. Bring it to a boil. After the first water boils, pour and rinse the beans in a colander.

Place the beans back into the pot and add enough water to cover the beans. Boil the beans until ¾ cooked, approximately 30 minutes. Rinse in colander.

Remember, if using canned beans make sure to rinse them first.

Place the beans into the pot. Add the onions, garlic, carrots, and celery to the beans. Add enough water to *almost* cover the beans. When the pot begins to boil add the tomatoes, basil leaves, salt, and pepper to taste AND turn the flame down to low. Simmer. Check continuously so they don't burn. When almost done, add olive oil, stir, and serve hot.

Great alone or with black or brown rice. This is an old vegetarian dish from Kardamyla, Chios passed down from my Gia Gia (grandmother) Maria. My mother would make this when we were fasting for Easter.

Demme's Healthier Dolmades (Grape Leaves)

1 16 oz. jar of tender, store bought grapevine leaves

3 large onions chopped

½ cup of avocado oil

½ cup of olive oil

2 cups of rice (½ cup of black rice, ½ cup of brown rice, ½ cup of quinoa, ½ cup *Lundberg Wild Blend* Rice)

You can also just use *Lundberg Wild Blend* Rice all on its own.

2 cups of chopped fresh dill

2 tablespoons fresh mint, minced

Salt and pepper to taste

2 lemons, juice only

Water as needed

1 heaping tablespoon of tomato paste or 1 cup of fresh tomatoes crushed

Note: *For the regular version use white rice and only olive oil.*

If possible, buy the prepared grapevine leaves and rinse lightly with cold water. Cut the stems from each leaf with scissors. Toss them in a pot of boiling water for 2 minutes until the leaves soften just a little. Remove and spread on a platter, let cool. Set aside 3 leaves for placing on top of the rolled dolmades.

To prepare the filling, sauté the chopped onion in avocado oil until lightly golden in color. Add the rice and let it cook for 2-3 minutes so the rice picks up the flavor of the onion. Add tomato paste or 3 tomatoes, the dill, salt, pepper, and mint. Also add 3 cups of water to the rice and stir. Cook using a low flame, stirring constantly, until the rice is about ¾ of way cooked. This will take about 15 minutes.

When filling the leaves, keep the shiny side of the leaf on the outside. Lay the leaves flat, then put one teaspoonful of the filling close to the stem area of the leaf.

Fold the stem area of the leaf over the rice mixture. Bring up both sides of the leaf and lay them over the rice mixture. Start rolling the dolmade, like rolling a cigarette/cigar. Place the stuffed leaves in a pot, open side down so they don't open when they swell up during the cooking process.

Lay them in even and tight rows. When 1 layer is complete, make a second layer Continue layering until you have finished all the rice mixture. Place the 3 leaves you have set aside, on top of the dolmades.

Place a small plate on top of the leaves. This will keep your dolmades from opening while cooking. Add enough water to the pot to cover the stuffed leaves, then add lemon juice to the water. Cover the pot and cook on low heat until the liquid has been absorbed. This should take about 45 minutes. Enjoy these alone with some tzatziki sauce as a side dish or as an appetizer. Greeks also eat it with Greek yogurt. Enjoy!!

Salad & Soup Recipes

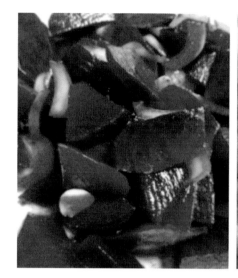 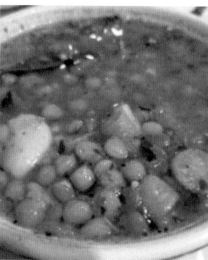 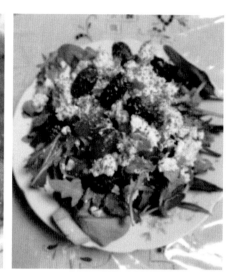

Fasolada Salad
(Black Eyed Pea Salad)

Nistisimi Salad
(Greek Potato Salad)

Kardamylitissa
(Greek Salad Feta and Olives)

Himoniatiki
(Cabbage Salad with Lemon)

Tabouli

Cucumber Tomato Salad

Aunt Tina's Beets Salad

Panagiotis Horta- Dandelion Greens

Eugenia's Avgolemono Soup and
New Version with Kale

Gia Gia Anna's Lentil Soup

Recipes

Fasolada Salad

1 pound of black eyed peas dry or 2 cans of cooked black eyed peas

½ cup of olive oil

2 large fresh tomatoes cubed

1 large red onion sliced

1-2 Lemons squeezed (depending how much lemon you like)

2 tablespoons of Bragg Apple Cider Vinegar

1 cup of chopped parsley

1-2 medium cucumbers cubed

A handful of black olives pitted and chopped

Salt and pepper to taste

Oregano to taste

Red cracked pepper (optional)

If using dry beans, soak overnight then rinse in am. Put in pot with enough water to cover them and cook on low to medium heat until tender. Watch to make sure there is always enough water so they don't stick. When done, rinse well.

Put all ingredients in a bowl and mix. Let stand in fridge until served. The longer in fridge the better the taste.

Nistisimi (Greek potato salad)

1 Pound of red potatoes boiled and cubed (larger cubes)

1 large firm tomato cubed

1 lemon squeezed

1 cup of parsley chopped

1 green bell pepper cubed

1 large red onion chopped

¼ cup of Bragg Apple Cider Vinegar

Handful of kalamata black olives chopped or whole your preference

Salt and pepper to taste

Oregano to taste

Red cracked pepper to taste (optional)

Put everything in a glass bowl and stir well. Let stand in fridge for 30 minutes until ready to serve. Enjoy!!

Kardamylitissa

(Greek Salad Feta and Olives)

1 head of romaine lettuce chopped sliced to your liking or 2 handfuls of mixed greens, arugula or watercress

2 large ripe but firm tomatoes sliced

2 medium cucumber sliced

1 large red onion sliced

Handful of kalamata black olives

1 large green bell pepper

½ pound of coarsely crumbled firm feta cheese

Oregano to taste

Salt and pepper to taste

½ cup olive oil

¼ cup Bragg Apple Cider Vinegar

Place chopped lettuce in a large salad bowl. Add cucumbers, tomatoes, and onions. Put feta cheese, green peppers, and olives on top. Sprinkle with oregano. If making ahead of time, do not add salt and pepper or oil and vinegar until ready to serve. I don't usually add salt because the olives have enough salt for me.

Note: *Normally lettuce is usually not served in traditional Greek salads. On my journey to getting healthy I have learned that the more leafy greens I add to my meals the more my sugar levels improve.*

So healthy and happy eating!

Himoniatiki (Cabbage Salad with Lemon)

½ head of green or purple cabbage sliced

2 cups of shredded carrots

½ cup of Olive oil

2 lemons squeezed

Garlic powder to taste

Salt and pepper to taste

Bragg Apple Cider Vinegar

Put all ingredients together and mix well. Serve in about 20-30 minutes after mixing together. You will love this and so will your microbiome. Healthy and happy gut! Your loved ones will be begging you for this one quite often.

Tabouli Ala Greek

3 cups of Fresh parsley finely chopped

1 large tomato very cubed

1 medium cucumber cubed

1 red onion chopped

1 Lemon squeezed

Handful of kalamata olives sliced

½ cup of Olive oil

3 tablespoons of Bragg Apple Cider Vinegar

Make sure to chop all veggies very fine for this recipe. The pieces don't have to be small in order to achieve a great taste. I myself have cut the veggies a bit larger many times and the taste is still there. So have fun and enjoy!!

Mix all ingredients together and put in fridge until ready to serve. I put a Greek and healthier twist on this as you are supposed to use extra fine bulgur. I decided to take it out as we all know we get enough carbs throughout the day. Why add more?

Cucumber Tomato Salad

2 cucumbers sliced

2 tomatoes sliced

Oregano to taste

Salt and pepper to taste

Olive oil

Bragg Apple Cider Vinegar

Mix all ingredients together 10-15 minutes before serving.

Aunt Tina's Beets Salad

2 bunches of organic beets with beet greens

½ cup of olive oil

Red or yellow onion sliced

4 garlic cloves chopped

½ cup of Bragg Apple Cider Vinegar

Salt and pepper to taste

Cut stems off of beet bulbs. Wash well by scrubbing. No need to peel beet bulbs (my mom's trick.) Cut stems into 3 parts: lower stems, mid stems, and top leafy area. Put them all into one of two pots. Then fill both pots with water, add salt to give taste to the beet bulbs or beet greens.

Beet Bulbs: Boil for 60 minutes. When the beet bulbs are tender, cool them with cold water. The skins should peel off easily by just putting the cooked beets under running water and rubbing with fingers. Slice cooked beets thinly or however you prefer and put into a glass bowl. Add onions, garlic, olive oil, vinegar, salt, and pepper. Place in the fridge for about 30 minutes.

Beet Greens: Start boiling the greens when you put the beets in the fridge to cool. Cook until tender. The greens usually take about 30 minutes to cook. When done, put the greens in a glass bowl. Add salt and pepper, olive oil and vinegar. Cover until ready to eat.

Serve as two separate side dishes or mix them together. Both go great with fish, or chicken or red meat. Can be served with tzatziki or as an appetizer.

Panagioti's Horta- Dandelion Greens

2 bunches dandelion greens washed and chopped

½ cup of olive oil

2 Lemons squeezed

Salt and pepper to taste

Wash dandelion greens in a bowl a few times and throw out water each time. Chop into 3 parts; stems, mid stems, and leafy tops. Put a large pot of water on stove add salt and bring to a boil. Add the chopped dandelion stems first, then put the mid stems and leafy tops into the pot. Bring to a boil and cook until tender. Usually takes about 20 minutes. Drain and put into a glass bowl. When ready, serve with olive oil, lemon, and just a little more salt to taste if needed. Goes great with any protein or appetizer or salad. Great for your liver!

Eugenia's Avgolemono Soup and New Version with Kale

5 whole eggs beaten

6 Lemons squeezed juice only

1 whole chicken

2 cup of sliced carrots

6 stalks of celery whole

6 whole cloves of garlic

2 whole onions cut in half

3 whole bay leaves

Salt and pepper

Option 1:

1 cup of orzo from my mom's original recipe

Option 2:

7 whole Kale leaves, cut in quarters or 2 cups of spinach

Wash chicken and cut into quarters. Fill pot up with water. Add chicken, salt, pepper, bay leaves, onions, carrots, celery, and garlic. Boil until fully cooked, about 60 minutes. Then take chicken and veggies out of the pot. Put in baking pan. Sprinkle chicken with salt, pepper, oregano, paprika, and garlic. Set aside until 20 minutes before serving.

Strain chicken stock and put in a clean pot. At this time you must decide if you want use orzo, kale or spinach. If you chose orzo, put it in the chicken stock and bring to a boil. Shut off flame from stock. In a glass bowl, beat the eggs very well. Slowly add the lemon juice to the eggs, beating them constantly. Then pour a ladle spoon or two of stock into egg and lemon juice mixture. Stir well so the eggs don't clump/cut. When done, pour into the pot while continuously stirring.

Note: *Do not cover pot, it will cut/clump the eggs! If using spinach or kale instead of orzo, drop it into the pot and let it wilt.*

When the soup is done, let stand uncovered until ready to eat. Put chicken in broiler. Cook until golden brown, which usually takes about 7- 10 minutes. Enjoy with black pepper!

Gia Gia Anna's Lentil Soup

1 pound of brown lentils cleaned

4 stalks of chopped celery

2 cups of sliced carrots

2 chopped onion

8 Whole garlic cloves

2 Fresh tomatoes grated

Salt and pepper to taste

3 whole bay leaves

½ cup of avocado oil

Italian seasoning to taste

Optional: My favorite is red cracked pepper and apple cider vinegar.

Put lentils in a pot with enough water to cover them. Bring to a boil. Drain in a colander, thus throwing out the first water. This will reduce the gas one can experience from eating lentils and makes the lentils easier to digest. Put the lentils back into the pot. Add the onions, celery, carrots, bay leaves, salt, and pepper. Refill the pot with enough water to cover everything. Bring to a boil. Add tomatoes, garlic, and avocado oil. Cook on low heat and simmer until lentils are fully cooked. Serve hot with red cracked pepper to taste. An old Chios (island in Greece) favorite is to add some vinegar.

Entrée Recipes

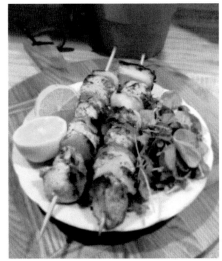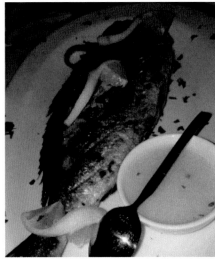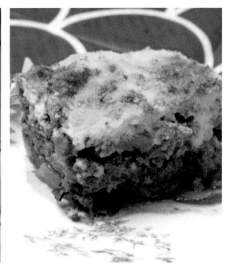

Keftedakia

Chicken Oreganato

Essam's Stuffed Tsipoura (Porgies)

Gia Gia Maria's Revithia

Kebobs

Fasolakia Ala Anna

Salmon Ala Demetra

Moussaka

Pastitsio

Recipes

Keftedakia

2 Pounds of chopped lean Beef, Turkey, Chicken, Veal or Lamb

(Your preference)

2 Large onions chopped

2 cups chopped parsley

4 cloves of fresh garlic minced

Fresh mint thinly chopped to taste

Oregano to taste

Salt and pepper to taste

¼ cup avocado oil

Put all ingredients in a mixing bowl. Mix everything together just enough to get all ingredients into meat. Then grease your hands and start shaping mixture into patties or meatballs. Lay in a baking pan and sprinkle lightly with salt, pepper, paprika, and oregano. Broil on one side until golden brown. Then broil on the other side. These cook very fast on broil so make sure you keep an eye on them. Your family will think you fried them.

Chicken Oreganato

1 whole Chicken quartered into pieces. This recipe serves 4-5 people. Depending on how many people you'll be serving, you may need more. I am Greek so we always have lots of food cooking just in case someone comes for dinner.

Oregano

2 Lemons squeezed juice only

4-5 Garlic cloves minced

¼ cup Avocado oil

6- 8 medium red potatoes with skin quartered

Salt and pepper to taste

Place the cut up potatoes in a large baking pan. Add salt, pepper, oregano, and oil. Mix to get the flavor and spices everywhere. Then lay chicken pieces, side down, on top of the potatoes or mixed in with them. Add the lemon juice. Pour in enough water to cover the potatoes. Put in the oven and bake at 475° F for about 20 minutes or until chicken is golden brown. Remove from oven and turn the chicken over. Let cook a bit more to get chicken golden brown on top. This should take about 10-15 minutes depending on your oven. Then check to see if potatoes are cooked and chicken is done. If not, cook a bit more. You may need to add a little more water. Potatoes soak up a lot of water when cooking. Also be careful not to use too much water. Serve hot with a salad or cooked veggies.

Essam's Stuffed Tsipoura (Whole Porgies)

4 fresh Porgies (fish) cleaned (gutted) and scaled

* Depending how many people will be served you may need more.

Oregano

½ bunch of parsley

2 Green bell peppers

4 cloves of garlic

1 medium onion

Red cracked pepper

Cumin to taste

Salt and pepper to taste

Clean and scale the fish. Using a knife and make a slit on each side of the fish bellies. Salt and pepper then lay in baking pan. Put all ingredients except oregano in food processor and mix well. Take mixture and stuff the porgies/fish bellies from underneath, using the opening from gutting the fish.

Put stuffed porgies on baking sheet. Sprinkle with oregano and cook in oven on broil. Cook for 7-10 minutes, then turn over to cook on the other side until golden brown. Serve with lemon slices, beet salad, Panagiotis Horta (dandelions) and a prepared rice dish or potatoes.

This is a very heart healthy meal and a great way to add protein to one's diet!

Gia Gia Maria's Revithia (Healthier Version)

1 can of chickpeas or dry chick peas

2 onions chopped

2 fresh tomatoes or 1 can of diced tomatoes

1 tablespoon of butter

1 cup of brown rice

½ cup of quinoa

1 cup of black rice

3 cloves of garlic minced

1 cup of chopped parsley

2 Tablespoons avocado oil

Put the butter in a pot and melt. Then add the brown rice, quinoa, and black rice to the pot, stir into the butter on a medium flame. Add 7 cups of water, salt and pepper to taste. Stir the contents of the pot. When it starts to boil, cover and put on a very low flame for 15- 20 minutes or until rice mixture is cooked. (You may need more water or longer time for everything to be fully cooked.)

Check on rice often because it will absorb water and can easily burn. Stir frequently towards the end of the cooking process. In another pot, sauté the onions and garlic in the avocado oil until golden brown. Add the chickpeas, tomatoes, parsley, salt, and pepper. Cook on medium heat.

*If using canned chickpeas this dish will be done in 15 minutes.

After rice is cooked, serve chickpeas on top. You can add cracked red pepper for a spicy twist. So good all by itself. This is a very healthy dish for your microbiome and gut health! Enjoy!

Note: *If you prefer to use white rice, use 2½ cups.*

Kebobs

Choose A Meat of Your Preference...

Lamb shoulder cut into cubes or

Chicken breast cubed or

Beef cubed

2 Purple onions quartered

1 red pepper cut into large pieces

1 green pepper cut into large pieces

1 yellow pepper cut into large pieces

5 cloves of garlic minced

3 Lemons squeezed juice only

2 Green peppers sliced in larger pieces to fit on stick

Paprika

½ cup of olive oil

Oregano to taste I prefer lots but that is up to you

Salt and pepper to taste

Choose the meat you want to use. The night before you will put ½ of the lemon juice, garlic, olive oil, paprika, oregano, salt, and pepper into a bowl with the meat of your choice. Cover and put in fridge to marinate overnight. The next day you will use kebab sticks and put the marinated meat and veggies on the sticks. Alternate between veggies and meat. Start the grill. BBQ on all four sides of the meat until there are grill marks on all sides. Make sure to not overcook if it's chicken. Pour the remaining lemon over the meat before serving. If you really want to feel like you are in Greece, do this next step: In a small bowl add the remaining lemon juice and some olive oil, oregano, salt, and pepper. Stir well and pour over meat. YUM!!

Note: You may also do this in a skillet with no sticks. Great with tzatziki and salad or over rice or as a sandwich on pita bread. *OPA!!*

Fasolakia Ala Anna

2 pounds of fresh string beans washed and cleaned of stems

Or 2 bags of frozen organic string beans

2 cups of sliced carrots

3 medium red potatoes

2 onions chopped

2 fresh tomatoes grated or 1 can of diced tomatoes

½ bunch of parsley chopped

1 tbsp of avocado oil

2 Tablespoons of olive oil

4 bay leaves

Oregano, salt and pepper to taste

In a large pan, sauté onions with avocado oil until onions are clear. Add carrots and string beans. Sauté for 5 minutes, just enough to get the flavor into the beans and carrots. Add the potatoes, salt, pepper, oregano, and bay leaves. Fill the pot with just enough water to almost cover the contents of the pot. Put flame on medium to low. Do not cover. Let cook for about 20 minutes or until everything is tender to your liking. When almost done, drop parsley and olive oil into the pot and stir well. At this time, check to see if the carrots and potatoes are done. Serve hot as a side or all by itself.

Note: *Many Greeks like to make this with beef. If you prefer to add meat start with the beef cubed. Boil for 20 minutes with salt and pepper and 1 whole onion.*

After this is done, throw out the onion and pour the water down the drain. Sauté the meat with the chopped onions and move onto the rest of the steps above. Enjoy with the family! Great dish for winter.

Salmon Ala Demetra

6 pieces of salmon

Fresh dill or dry dill

Salt and pepper to taste

Cracked red pepper (optional)

Paprika

Lemon wedges

¼ cup of avocado oil or olive oil

Set oven to broil. Oil the pan and lay the sliced salmon on the pan, skin side down. Sprinkle salt, pepper, paprika, and dill on all pieces. You can also add cracked red pepper if you like it spicy. Cook in broiler until golden brown or for about 10-15 minutes. To check if ready, put a fork in middle of fish and twist slightly. If flakey, it is ready. Garnish with lemon wedges. Enjoy with dandelion greens or beets or some tzatziki or a Greek salad.

Demme's Healthy Moussaka

4 - 5 large Idaho or russet potatoes cleaned and sliced round

2 large onions chopped

4 -6 cloves of garlic

1 ½ pounds of beef chopped

½ bunch of fresh parsley

4 medium zucchini thinly sliced lengthwise

4 eggplant thinly sliced lengthwise

2 large tomatoes grated or 1 can of diced tomatoes

Oregano, Salt and pepper to taste

3-4 Bay leaves

¼ cup of olive oil (your preference)

Or a few sprays of avocado oil just enough so onion doesn't stick to pan

Or no oil and just use a little of water

Demme's Healthier Bechamel sauce

8 tablespoons of organic butter

8-10 heaping tablespoons of fine coconut flour

2 heaping tablespoons of arrowroot flour

4-5 cups of mixture of unsweetened hemp milk, coconut milk, cashew milk or almond milk

2 whole eggs

Salt and pepper to taste

Step 1: Preheat oven to 475° F. Prepare your ingredients for the Moussaka recipe above. On a baking sheet with parchment paper, lay zucchini and eggplant slices close together. Salt and pepper them and cook lightly until lightly browned. Turnover and do the same on the other side. Continue this until you finish all zucchini and eggplant. While these are cooking, lightly spray or grease a large baking pan. Lay raw potatoes on the bottom of the pan. Salt and pepper to taste. Then begin to layer the zucchini and eggplant on top until you have transferred them all over. Set aside until you are done with the next step.

Step 2: In a large frying pan, sauté chopped onions and garlic in avocado oil for a few minutes until golden color. Add chopped beef and continue to sauté. Stir and let meat cook until browned. This usually takes about 10-15 minutes on medium heat. Begin to add spices: salt and pepper, oregano and bay leaves. Cook for 5 minutes and then add tomatoes and chopped parsley. Continue to cook for 5-10 minutes more. You may need to add a little water at this time. Let cook 1 minute more. Pour all meat contents on top of zucchini and eggplant layers in baking pan. Set aside until last steps are completed.

Step 3: In a large saucepan, *using the healthier bechamel sauce recipe above*, melt the butter on a low flame. When fully melted, slowly add the coconut flour blending thoroughly. Cook for 1 minute, stirring constantly. On low heat, begin to slowly add the dairy free milk. Stir with a wooden spoon until the mixture thickens and is a creamy sauce. Turn off the flame on stove and set pot with creamy sauce aside. In a small cup, add a few tablespoons of room temperature dairy free milk with the arrowroot flour in it. Mix well and pour into the creamy sauce in the pot. Stir for a few minutes more until the consistency is perfect! In another small bowl, beat the eggs well. Add the salt and pepper, stir until blended. Slowly add the egg mixture to the cream sauce and blend in the cream. When done, you should have a very creamy sauce to pour on top of the moussaka. Add grated almond cheese or dairy free cheeses or regular cheese if you prefer.

Step 4: Pour the bechamel sauce on top of everything. Make sure to spread it out evenly as you pour. If you prefer, sprinkle gluten free breadcrumbs on top before baking. Put in preheated oven at 475° F for about 35 - 40 minutes or until golden brown on top. Let the moussaka cool for about 20 minutes before serving.

Enjoy your Healthy Moussaka!! *With this recipe you have cut out saturated fat and unneeded carbs while adding in healthier nutrients for your body! The taste is soooo close to the real one you won't even notice….OPA!*

My Mother's Moussaka—Original Recipe

4 - 5 large Idaho or russet potatoes cleaned and sliced round

2 large onions chopped

4 -6 cloves of garlic

1 ½ pounds of beef chopped

½ bunch of fresh parsley

4 medium zucchini thinly sliced lengthwise

4 eggplant thinly sliced lengthwise

2 large tomatoes grated or 1 can of diced tomatoes

3 cups of grated Kefalograviera Cheese or Pecorino Romano

Oregano, Salt and pepper to taste

3-4 Bay leaves

¼ cup of olive oil

Original Bechamel Sauce

8 tablespoons of butter

10-12 tablespoons of flour

5 cups of milk at room temperature

2 eggs

3 tablespoons of breadcrumbs for top

Salt and pepper to taste

Step 1: Clean and peel potatoes. Cut into round pieces and fry. Then set in bottom of baking tray when done. Set aside and continue with next step.

Step 2: Stir fry the onions and garlic in a frying pan until golden in color. Then put chopped meat in pan and break up with a fork. While the meat is being browned begin to put the salt, pepper, oregano, parsley, and bay leaves into the mixture. When everything has cooked, toss in the tomatoes. Cook for a few more minutes. When done, make sure to pull out the bay leaves and discard them.

Step 3: Fry all the veggies and set aside on a pile of paper towels in order to pull out the grease. In the baking pan, where the potatoes are, begin to layer the cooked veggies. Sprinkle each layer with grated cheese. Then place the cooked meat on top. Sprinkle another light layer of the grated cheese on top of the meat. Set aside until completing the next step.

Step 4: *Use the Original Bechamel Sauce recipe.* In a saucepan, melt the butter on low flame. When fully melted slowly add the flour, blending thoroughly. On low heat begin to slowly add the milk, mixing constantly. Stir until the mixture thickens. Turn off the burner and let stand. In another small bowl, beat the eggs well, then add the salt and pepper. Stir until blended. Slowly add egg mixture to the cream sauce. Add the remainder of the cheese.

Step 5: Pour bechamel sauce on top. Make sure to evenly spread the sauce over the top of everything. Sprinkle breadcrumbs on top and put into preheated oven. Bake at 475° F for about 35 - 40 minutes or until golden brown on top. Enjoy your Original Moussaka!! This recipe comes from my mother. I believe it is from Kardamyla, Chios. It was my Gia Gia Maria's recipe with influences from many generations of women on that side of the family.

Demme's Healthier Pastitsio

1 package of brown rice pasta (I prefer Pasta Joy)

3 large yellow onions chopped

5 -6 cloves of garlic minced

1 ½ pounds of beef chopped

1 bunch of parsley chopped

3-4 whole Bay leaves

Oregano, salt and pepper

2 large whole fresh tomatoes or 1 can of diced tomatoes

¼ cup of olive oil or avocado oil your preference

Demme's Healthier Bechamel Sauce

8 tablespoons of organic butter

8-10 heaping tablespoons of fine coconut flour

2 heaping tablespoons of arrowroot flour

4-5 cups of mixture of unsweetened hemp milk, coconut milk, cashew milk or almond milk

2 whole eggs

Salt and pepper to taste

Step 1: Boil pasta according to directions on bag. Let stand in covered pot with no flame, for about 10 minutes. Place in colander and rinse with cold water. Put into a deep dish pan, the size of a lasagna pan. Sprinkle the cooked pasta with shredded vegan cheese, oregano, salt, and pepper. Drizzle 2 tablespoons of avocado oil onto the pasta mixture and stir.

Step 2: In a large frying pan, sauté chopped onions and garlic in avocado oil for a few minutes until golden in color. Then put the chopped beef in pan and sauté. Stir and let cook until meat is browned. This usually takes about 10-15 minutes on medium heat. Begin to add spices: salt, pepper, oregano, and bay leaves. Cook for 5 minutes and then add tomatoes and chopped parsley. Cook for 5-10 minutes more. You may need to add a little water at this time and let cook for another minute. When done, take out bay leaves and throw them away. Pour all meat contents on top of pasta in baking pan. Let stand until last steps are completed.

Step 3: *Use the Healthier Bechamel Sauce recipe.* In a large saucepan, melt the butter on low flame. When fully melted, slowly stir in the coconut flour blending thoroughly. Let cook for 1 minute stirring constantly. On low heat, begin to slowly add the dairy free milk. Stir with wooden spoon until the mixture thickens and is a creamy sauce. Turn off the flame and set pot with cream sauce aside. In a small cup, add a few tablespoons of room temperature dairy free milk with the arrowroot flour. Mix well and pour into the cream sauce in the pot. Stir for a few minutes more until the consistency is perfect! In another small bowl, beat the eggs well. Add the salt and pepper, stir until blended. Slowly add egg mixture to the cream sauce and blend with cream. When done, you should have a very creamy sauce to put on top of pastitsio. If you would like, you may add grated almond cheese or dairy free cheeses or regular cheese if you prefer. Sprinkle with breadcrumbs and cook on middle shelf in 475° F degree oven for 30-40 minutes or until golden brown. When done, let stand for 20 minutes before serving. Serve with a Greek salad and enjoy!

Aunt Tina's Pastitsio

Original Bechamel topping

1 package of Misko Pastitsio Macaroni or 1 ½ packages of elbows or penne

8 tablespoons of butter

10 - 12 heaping tablespoons of all-purpose flour

5 cups of milk at room temperature

2 eggs

3 cups of grated Kefalograviera Cheese or Pecorino Romano Cheese

3 tablespoons of breadcrumbs for top

Salt and pepper to taste

Step 1: Boil pasta according to directions on bag then let stand in covered pot with no flame for about 10 minutes. In a colander, drain the pasta. Put the cooked pasta into a deep dish pan, the size of a lasagna pan. Sprinkle cheese, oregano, salt, and pepper. Stir together.

Step 2: In a large frying pan, sauté the chopped onions and garlic in avocado oil. Continue until golden in color. Add chopped beef and continue to sauté until meat is browned. This usually takes about 10-15 minutes on medium heat. Begin to add spices: salt and pepper, oregano and bay leaves. Cook for 5 minutes and then add tomatoes and chopped parsley. Cook for 5-10 minutes more. When meat is done, take out bay leaves and discard. Pour all meat contents on top of pasta, making an even layer across the baking pan. Let stand until last steps are completed.

Step 3: *Use the Original Bechamel Sauce recipe.* In a saucepan, melt the butter on low flame. When fully melted add the flour slowly to the melted butter, blending thoroughly. On low heat begin to slowly add the milk, mixing constantly. Stir until the mixture thickens. Shut fire off and let stand. In another small bowl, beat the eggs well. Add the salt and pepper, stir until well blended. Slowly add egg mixture to the cream sauce. Add the remainder of cheese. When done you should have a very creamy sauce to pour on top of your Pastitsio. Sprinkle with breadcrumbs and cook on middle shelf in 475° F oven for 30-40 minutes or until golden brown.

When done, let it cool off for about 20 minutes before serving. Serve with a Greek salad and enjoy!

Dessert Recipes

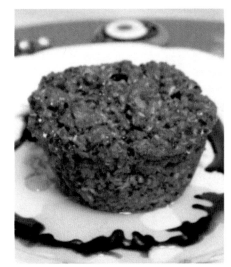 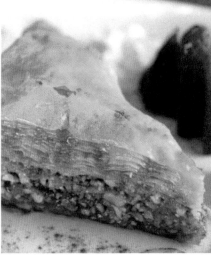 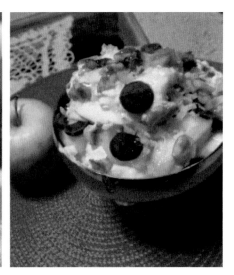

Baklava Quinoa Muffin

Baklava Ala Demme
(The REAL Greek Baklava)

Karidopita Ala Eugenia

Greek Yogurt Parfait Ala Adam

Recipes

Baklava Quinoa Muffin

Ingredients for about 18-20 muffins depending on muffin trays used:

3 eggs

4 ripe medium bananas

3/4 cup coconut oil

4 cups cooked quinoa

1 cup almond or coconut flour

10 packets of monk fruit in the raw and 2 tbsp honey

3 tbsp cinnamon

1 tsp allspice or ground cloves (optional)

3 tsp baking powder

½ cup almond milk, coconut or hemp milk (add tbsps of milk if batter is too thick or dry)

1 cup of unsweetened coconut flakes or shredded coconut

1 cup of raw chopped walnuts for mixture save a few for garnish

1 cup of raw whole almonds for mixture save a few for garnish

And or ½ cup unsweetened dark chocolate or stevia sweetened chips (optional)

or 1 cup blueberries (frozen or raw) optional

STEPS

1. Set oven to 375° F

2. Mix eggs, banana, and coconut oil together in bowl.

3. Then add remaining ingredients, except for the blueberries (if using them.) Mix thoroughly with a wooden mixing spoon or rubber spatula.

4. Toss in the blueberries and stir. (blueberries are optional)

5. Use paper cupcake/muffin cups. Set them into the muffin pan. Then pour the batter into the cups. Add nuts on top for a garnish. (optional)

6. Bake for 30 minutes at 375° F. Then turn up the temperature to 400° F, set timer for 5 minutes (depending on oven it may need a little more time than the extra 5 min.) Cook until golden brown.

Tips to make it even better!!. Slice off the top of a muffin. Place the top and bottom in a toaster that can handle bagels or place on a cookie sheet and broil in the oven. Once hot, spread with nut butter or organic butter. Add a light drizzle of raw honey (honey is optional). These muffins are a perfect treat for breakfast and also make a great 'on the go' snack.

Baklava Ala Demme (The REAL Greek Baklava)

2 cups of almonds chopped

2 ½ cups of walnuts chopped

1 ½ tablespoon cinnamon

1 tsp of ground clove

1 ½ cups of melted butter

1 Package of Phyllo dough

The Syrup

4 cups of sugar

3 cups of water

2 pieces of stick cinnamon

6 cloves

1 whole lemon squeezed and peel

Mix together the chopped nuts, cinnamon, and ground clove powder. Brush butter on a cookie sheet pan. Lay 1st sheet of phyllo on the pan, to create the bottom layer. As you pile the phyllo sheets, brush each sheet with butter. Do this for 6 sheets. Sprinkle some of the nut mixture onto the 6th sheet. Now alternate a sheet of phyllo with nuts on top of each sheet. Make sure to butter the phyllo before adding the nuts. Continue doing this until you run out of nut mixture. Then add 6 phyllo sheets, buttering as you go. Trim any sheets if hanging over pan. At this time push down on the whole thing to make sure it is compacted. Score the baklava into diamond shaped pieces or squares, your preference. Wet your fingers and shake them over the top of the baklava. Bake on middle shelf in preheated, 250° F oven for about 1 hour or until top is golden brown.

*A good way to check that it is fully done is to take the baklava out of oven and slip a knife or spatula under the bottom layer, lift to make sure the bottom layer is golden brown. Take out of the oven and let cool.

To prepare the syrup put the sugar and water in pot to boil. Add the cinnamon sticks, cloves, and lemon juice. Drop the whole peel in the water. Let that cook on the stove for about 10 minutes on a low flame. When the baklava has had time to cool, pour the hot syrup over the top. Let it stand for a few minutes and then cut through to the bottom layers, following the score marks on the top.

Note: Always pour hot over cold, never hot on hot (this will not affect the flavor, yet it will make the baklava soggy.) Baklava must always be crisp and moist at the same time. Enjoy!! This recipe originally had more sugar, which I have reduced since getting it into my own hands. I also have reduced the butter and changed the nuts to be both almonds and walnuts for more protein and extra crunch. Enjoy with an espresso or frappe.

Karidopita Ala Eugenia

½ cup of butter

4 eggs, separated

¾ cup of cognac

3 cups walnuts

1 ½ cups of toasted breadcrumbs (use gluten free bread, if you'd like)

1 ½ tsp of baking powder

1 tablespoon cinnamon

The syrup

2 cups of water

2 cups of sugar (optional)

1 lemon rind

1 piece of cinnamon stick

Whip the butter until light in color. In a separate bowl, beat the egg yolks until thick. Add sugar, beating in thoroughly. Add the mixture to the butter and continue to beat until well blended. Mix in the cognac, then add the walnuts.

Mix the breadcrumbs with the baking powder and cinnamon. Beat the egg whites until stiff. Fold breadcrumbs and egg whites into the batter. Stir gently. Pour into a buttered baking pan or mold. Bake in a preheated 350° F oven on the middle shelf for about an hour. Remove from the oven and cool partially. If in a mold, turn out onto a platter once cooled.

In the meantime, start preparing the syrup. Put the water, sugar (optional), lemon, and cinnamon stick in a saucepan and bring to a boil. Boil for about 5 minutes. Remove the rind and cinnamon stick. Pour hot over the karithopita. Serve with coffee, tea or alone. Enjoy!!

Greek Yogurt Parfait Ala Adam

½ cup of Plain Greek yogurt

1 Handful of nuts of your choice

1 tsp Coconut flakes or shredded coconut

Cinnamon to taste

Honey

½ cup of fruit in season of your choice

In a bowl, put in the yogurt then sprinkle remaining ingredients on top. Sprinkle chocolate syrup or chocolate chips on top as well. Serve with a little dollop of whipped cream.

Note: This was and still is Adam's favorite dessert, next to ice cream or baklava. He has made it a dessert through lifestyle. I am super excited that he sees this as a snack, rather than snacking on unhealthy choices.

Drink Recipes

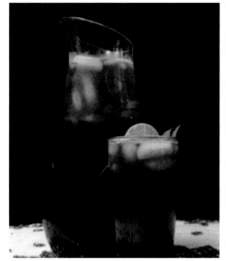 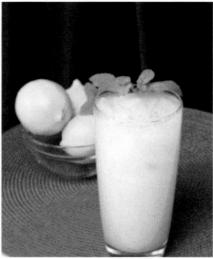 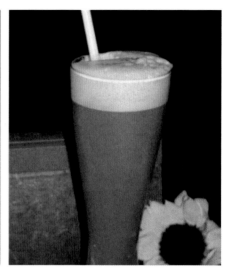

Gia Gia Anna's Chamomile

Demme Frappe

Lemon Mint

Mama Haga's Karkadea
(Hibiscus Drink)

Recipes

Gia Gia Anna's Chamomile

Boil enough water for the amount of people you want to serve. Add 1 tablespoon of fresh chamomile flowers or use a tea bag. Let boil for a few minutes on low. Pour into tea cups. Add lots of lemon and honey. Very beneficial for colds and for sleepless nights, anxiety, and stomach issues. This tea is a staple in all Greek homes, especially in Kardamyla, Chios.

Demme Iced Frappe (*with liquor or without, serve hot or cold*)

1 ½ Heaping Teaspoons Nescafe Classic—Frappe coffee

Sugar your preference

Milk or almond milk/coconut milk/water

Water (initially 1 tblsp of water)

Ice cubes

To Enjoy with Liquor: Add Kahlua or Baileys Irish cream your preference

In a shaker, put 1 tablespoon of water and the Nescafe Classic Instant Coffee. Sugar is optional. Shake constantly until you have a creamy substance. Pour in a glass with ice. Then add milk or water until the drink reaches the top. If you prefer liquor, add a shot or 2 of Bailey's Irish Cream or Kahlua! You can also add a sprinkle of cinnamon on top!

Lemon mint

1 whole lemon

20 oz of Water

Ice cubes

Fresh mint leaves about 10 leaves or 2 whole stems and leaves

Honey, sugar or Stevia to taste (Your preference)

Cut stem off of lemon. In a blender or processor add the whole lemon, pits and all. Also add water, mint, and your preference of sweetener. Blend until everything is in liquid form. If your blender doesn't get everything done, don't worry. Use a strainer to strain all liquid into glasses. Add ice and top with a mint leaf!! This drink is not only refreshing, your liver, and microbiome will thank you!

Mama Haga's Karkadea (Hibiscus Drink)

1 cup of dried Hibiscus flowers

6 cups of water

Rose water 1 tablespoon

1 whole lime sliced

Honey, Stevia, sugar to taste (Your Preference)

Put the water and hibiscus into a pot and bring to a boil. After boiling for 5 minutes, let stand for about 10 minutes in order to cool. Fill a pitcher with ice. Pour cooled drink into the pitcher. Put the rose water and slices of lime into the drink. Enjoy! Hibiscus helps to relax the body and is very calming. This drink comes from Alexandria, Egypt from my Mother-in-law's family.

About the Author

As a woman who has struggled with being overweight all of her life, Demme Matheos became her own hero. Her journey towards better health has been bitter sweet with many ups and downs. Raised in a Greek family with social gatherings being mainly around food and suffering from a metabolism disorder, Demme ended up at 330 pounds by 42 years old.

Losing her mother at age 47, Demme was only 15 years old, and experiencing what looked like a heart attack by age 42, Demme decided she did not want to leave her then 6 year old son motherless.

The week before she ended up in the hospital, she had bought a size 32 blouse and was about to buy an electric chair scooter.

For the past 4 years Demme has made an effort to not have weight loss as her focus. She teaches this mindset to her clients as well. Demme understands that focusing on bio-individuality is key. She is a certified IIN Health Coach who has also successfully completed the Gut Health Course, with expertise in understanding the fundamentals of both digestive and gut health. Demme understands the factors that can influence conditions of gut imbalance, as well as dietary and lifestyle choices that may promote optimal health.

Demme's doctor has given her the 'okay sign' to get off of her diabetes medications. This came about by eating healthy, moving more, and working on how she reacts to stress.

Each day Demme is learning new habits and seeing what works in her life.

This book has been on her mind for a few years now. Her family and friends have always told her that she is an amazing cook. Demme has been changing family recipes into more healthier versions since her hospitalization in 2010. She has also been testing them all out on her extended family. They especially love her Greek and Egyptian dishes that were passed down from family members. Demme has included many of those recipes in this book. They are made with healthy, nutritious foods that are great tasting and will not spike your sugar or insulin.

A Note From the Author

I would love to hear all about your experiences with changing your foods and tasting these recipes. Come by my website and write a review in the contact page and on Amazon. Also, have a look around for recommended products that I use to assist me in living healthier. www.RebootYourselfNow.com

Keep a look out for my next cookbook in THE HEALTHIER GREEK series, which will have great recipes that I have changed throughout my life. I have infused them with my Greek and Egyptian twists.

In this book, I share the knowledge I have gained and the recipes I have tweaked along with the baby steps I took to change behaviors that my doctors and I thought would NEVER change.

As I noted in the Dedication, this book is dedicated to many people including two amazing Doctors who have changed my life forever.

Once again I'd like to recognize Dr. David Wendell, whom I met in the beginning of my journey back in 2007 and Dr. George Kosmides who made a huge impact on my life in such a short time.

I thank you both for all your knowledge and I will forever remember your words. You both have helped me become the person I am today.

As I mentioned earlier, everything came to that life changing halt 8 years ago when I was admitted to the hospital on Mother's Day.

As you already know, my son Adam cried himself to sleep while I was away in the hospital. I felt so guilty and was determined to change. The diagnoses, especially the Type 2 Diabetes, scared the crap out of me.

When I got home, I tried everything in order to lower my fasting numbers. Instead of giving up, I started to change out a few unhealthy habits. I began to eat healthier, drink water, and I even started a walking routine.

Fast forward to 2016. I had finally lost 70 pounds and reduced my medications from 8 to 6. I plateaued for 2 years, despite all of my efforts. The dial on my scale wouldn't move and there were days that I just wanted to throw it in the garbage.

In fact, it was so easy to gain a few pounds by one little slip up, that it became harder and harder to lose more or even maintain the weight that I had already lost.

I've changed so many lifestyle habits since 2010. I knew my immune system was getting healthier because I wasn't sick all the time. My skin looked amazing and I felt great. I still had diabetes and I still took 2 medications. It was at this point that I started getting in touch with my body. I became aware of the signals my body was giving me, like letting me know when I was full or if I was hungry.

In November of 2017, I decided I would attempt to be a vegetarian. I pulled out all animal protein, except for eggs. I did feel a little bit better for a few days, however I also began to have a lot of spikes with my sugar levels. I knew something was wrong. After about a month I decided I just couldn't do it! I felt jittery and my blood sugar levels were not in control and I was constantly 'hangry'.

One thing Dr. George Kosmides taught me was 'to do what I can' each day, to pick

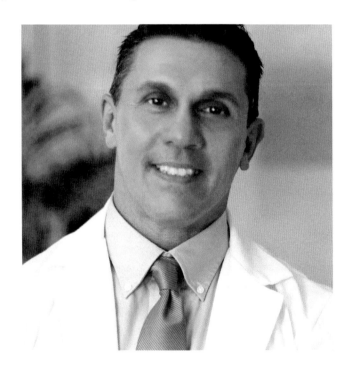

one thing that is doable. Something that will bring me closer to my goals.

He also advised me saying, "Once you have that down and you are consistent, add another. Do not overwhelm yourself with too many changes at once, because it will not become a habit." This is easily said and very hard to follow especially when you have an eating disorder and/or do not have healthy eating habits.

Let's be honest, if I had healthy eating habits I would not revolve my days around what I eat. For example, I would not be tempted to eat when I was bored, when I was happy, and celebratory, when I feel alone or overwhelmed. Through the 40 plus years of my life, food had become my best friend. I have now learned what affects my food choices. I had a second huge 'wakeup call' when one of my favorite cousins, Michael Sarris, passed away at age 54 .

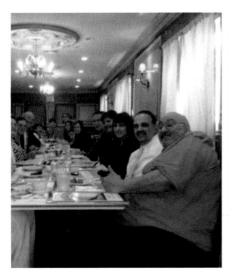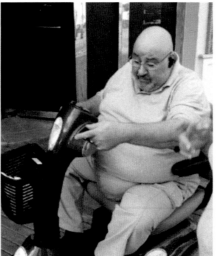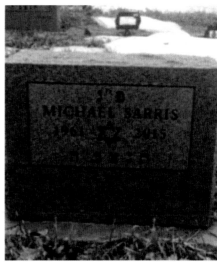

Each year I learned new things about myself and the habits that brought me closer to getting healthier each year.

When I got serious about getting healthy, the first thing that became apparent was that I didn't take care of myself. In fact I took care of everyone else first and if I made it on the list for the day or even week, I was lucky.

I committed to making sure that I did something every day for 60 minutes that brought me closer to my own health goals. Again, easier said than done! Then, I made sure that I had a plan and was prepared for anything. This one is still an issue, sometimes because life happens and sometimes I am not prepared. Which brings me to forgiving myself for slipping up from time to time. YOU CANNOT BE PERFECT!!

When I started in 2010, I was very unhealthy. I couldn't walk more than a few steps without being out of breath. In fact I was very scared because I had just gotten out of the hospital diagnosed with an Angina attack, COPD, Obesity, Type 2 Diabetes, High Cholesterol, Anxiety, Panic attacks, and Insomnia.

I tried to walk a few steps, but my breathing was awful. I was also uncomfortable having my picture taken.

When my son asked if he could take a picture of me, I felt I couldn't refuse him. This photo was taken from my deck days before I landed my butt in the hospital. After being hospitalized I got the both of us eating a healthier diet.

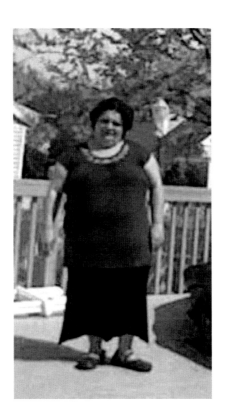
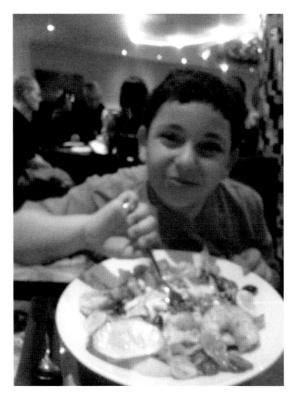

When I got out of the hospital I realized I needed help so I joined Weight Watchers. It was great because I had somewhere to start.

In the beginning I was forced to weigh myself, then sit in the meetings and listen to others who had the same issues with food as I did. It was great because I didn't feel alone anymore!

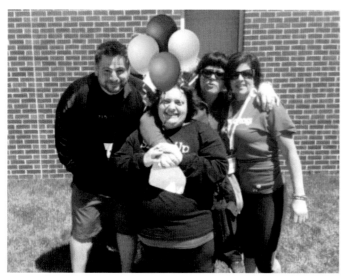 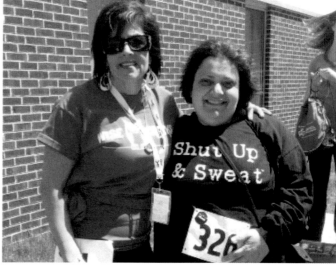

At that time my son and I started watching the reality show, The Biggest Loser. Mark Pinhasovich [left] lost 213 pounds while participating in the show. His cousin, Merav Landman-Fiorella, who is standing directly behind me with her arm over my shoulder, started at 289 and lost 134 pounds at home while Mark was away on the show. [right] Paulette Stallone and I. Paulette beat stage 4 colon cancer and this was her walk. She hosts this walk every year in Freehold, NJ. It is called the Colorectal Run Walk.

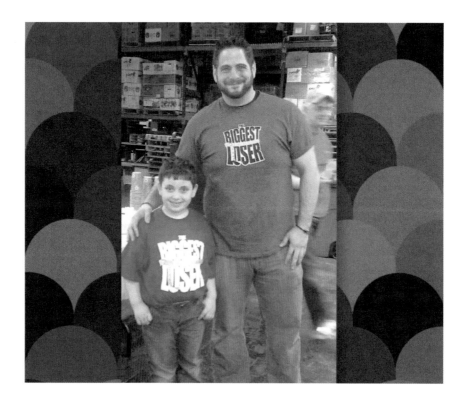

Adam Eliraky with Mark Pinhasovich

My son then 6 years old, started to join me once I had started my 10 minute walks. That's when I realized I had taught my son all my bad habits. Once I had worked up to a 15 minute walk, he was tired. That motivated me to do even more. [2010]

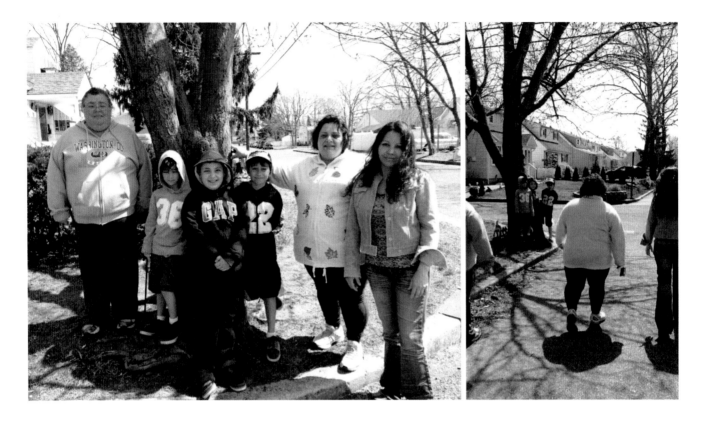

Walking with my son and the neighborhood gang!

I joined a gym and started doing light weights. I started to lose some weight and feel better.

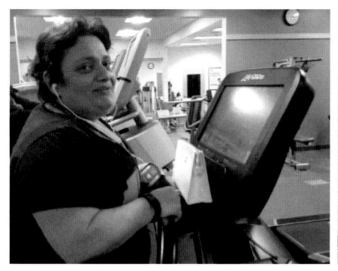
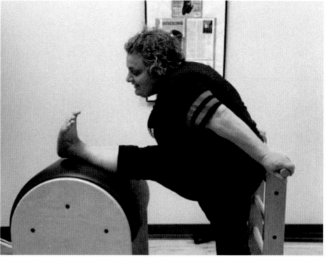

My depression, anxiety, and moodiness lifted when I went to the gym. So I wanted to go to the gym as often as I could. At some point I felt a lot better health wise and emotionally.

I was gradually taken off some medicines but I hit a plateau on the scale for months. I couldn't get it to move. I couldn't lose another pound for a while even though I was losing inches. Then, when I was finally feeling the best I had felt in years, tragedy hit and life happened!

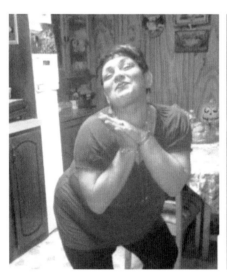
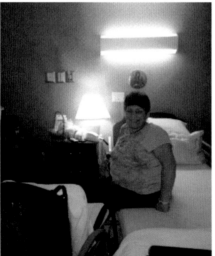
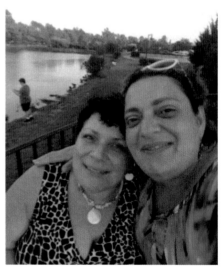

My sister had a severe stroke September 25, 2012, which left her paralyzed. About 2 months later my husband was involved in a severe car accident. That's when step one to getting healthier was lost AGAIN!! I forgot my goals, my dreams, my health, and myself!!!

Everything I had worked so hard for was gone. Fast forward 1 year later. I gained almost 40 pounds back. I stopped working out. Everything was almost back to where I had been when I started. I even had gotten off my diabetes meds and had to go back on again. I was sooooooo mad!

That's when I signed up to become an IIN Health Coach. It was the best decision I could have ever made for myself. As I studied, I realized that I had so much more to learn about taking care of my health. It wasn't only about the food. It was also about my mindset.

In my opinion it is crucial to all humans to feel they have achieved something in this lifetime. Living their life's purpose is huge but the sad truth is that so many of us get sucked into the hamster wheel of fortune and work, work, work with no awareness of our own enjoyments or dreams actually coming to fruition. We die without enjoying anything or feeling fulfilled.

Start today, get up and make a copy of the assessment sheet NOW! Print the MMC Self-Assessment from the Forms area of this book. Then fill it out so you can see where you need support. That way you can begin to start putting your focus on where you need it. The areas that are lower on the score are where you need to start focusing in order to feel like YOU AGAIN! As you begin to work on those areas, you will start to eat better and make better healthier choices. You will be amazed at the changes in mindset and the shifts that will happen in your life.

As you know, when I started, I made simple changes to my diet including cutting out MSG aka bouillon cubes and began to cook with coconut oil. I started buying more organic meats, fruits, and veggies. I started TO CURE MY IMMUNE SYSTEM by making these significant changes in my lifestyle habits.

I hit a plateau again in 2016. It was then that I 'happened' to be directed to a Periscope video by a Dr. George Kosmides. I didn't realize that this man would have such an impact on my life, but he did. As he talked about his program it sounded exactly like what I was already doing in my own life.

I had figured out that my body did very well on lower carbohydrates, good fats, and higher protein. The only thing different with his program was the timing of carbs and fruits. So I decided to try it out.

I joined his program and in 2 months I saw a huge difference in my blood sugar numbers. In seeing these results my general doctor at the time, wanted me to lower my diabetes medications. I was super excited and of course I couldn't wait to get off of them.

That's when everything went crazy AGAIN!

As soon as I went off that medicine, my sugar levels went out of whack. No one tells you this will happen when you reduce your meds. So, I fought with my high numbers for a while and then the shit hit the fan!!!!!!!

I started having continuous yeast infections for over 6 months. I never had them like this EVER!! It was horrible. My general doctor had done nothing but give me medicine, which did nothing for me. I cut as many carbs out of my diet as I could. I lowered my fruits to almost none!! I felt like I was back to where I had started! The worst thing is that my original goal of losing weight was halted once AGAIN!

Why? Because when your sugar spikes you cannot lose fat!

So once again, I was stuck at a plateau until my body decided to go into homeostasis, a place of synergistic balance known as good health.

That is when I decided to call my favorite doctor, Dr. David Wendel from Health and Wellness Center in Jackson, NJ.

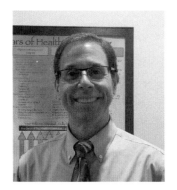

I vividly remember that particular conversation. I was just calling to say hello because we hadn't spoken in a few years. Then I decided to ask him this question, "Can you help me cure candida and chronic yeast infections?" He said, "Let's get you on the schedule for an initial consultation appointment!"

I started his protocol and 1 month later I ended up in the hospital with kidney stones. It had nothing to do with his protocol. My high levels of sugar had caused the kidney stones.

Fast forward to 2017 when I finally got rid of my yeast infections and all of my meds were lowered. I only had two Type 2 Diabetes medications left to go. So I continued my new lifestyle which at the time was high protein, high fiber, including veggies, low carbs, and almost no fruit because I had noticed that it spiked my sugar levels.

Like I have said from the beginning of this book: I AM NOT PERFECT and I am LEARNING MY OWN BODY as I MOVE FORWARD. Remember, EVERYONE IS DIFFERENT and YOUR BODY'S NEEDS CHANGE DAY BY DAY. You get to BECOME MINDFUL and LISTEN TO THE SIGNS of your OWN body. *Our bodies are amazing if given the chance to heal on their own.*

October 2017, I remember it well. I had decided to stay consistent with my exercise. I knew that the holidays were coming and I didn't want to go backwards. I had a tendency of gaining 15 pounds back every winter and then trying very hard to lose it again in the spring.

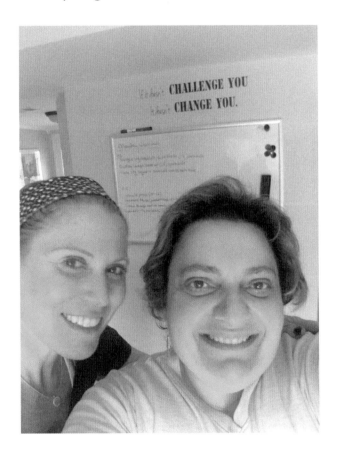

This time I hired a trainer to keep me accountable and at least keep my weight maintained through the winter months. I had learned that when I went to the gym I made better choices. This was a great investment for my health and I knew it would keep me accountable to reach my health goals sooner than later.

My trainer Amanda, pictured above, was a vegan and she tried very hard to get me to see the benefits of this type of diet. I did feel like my body needed a break from the animal proteins and was yearning for more vegetarian dishes. So I tried very hard to do it!

Although I felt great the first week, my body really just needed animal protein. My sugar levels went out of whack again and I couldn't stabilize them; so once again, I went back to my normal diet after about a month of yo-yoing. Many thanks to Amanda for inspiring me to add more vegan to this cookbook and for getting me to use the healthier recipes passed down in my family.

That was the last time that I got so sick that I needed antibiotics. As the year was ending and it was time for me to contemplate on what my focus would be for this year. My New Year's resolution for 2018 ended up being **mindfulness**.

Listening to My Body

Isn't that amazing? The person who always hated her body, her belly, is actually loving every part of it? Even her abdomen? I started listening to what it wanted. I started listening to my gut! I was feeling my whole body for the first time!!!!!!! In fact, as I did more of the mirror work and mindfulness exercises I realized that I hadn't been living IN MY OWN BODY FOR YEARS!!

Dr. George Kosmides', whose mission was to help as many diabetics as possible, had a great perspective concerning perfectionism…

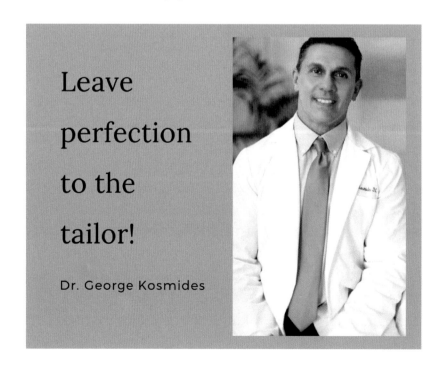

Leave perfection to the tailor!

Dr. George Kosmides

If you are not living your life to its fullest, something is holding you back and with mindfulness, kindness, and monitoring your thoughts on a daily basis you can get to the bottom of the issue.

As I mourned the loss of my friend and mentor, I continued to learn more about gut health, including my own gut. I began to incorporate even more, small yet significant changes into my life. And yet, it wasn't until I hit the unit in the Advanced Gut Health course at the Institute of Integrative Nutrition (IIN) which had to do with diabetes, obesity, and leaky gut that I finally realized the connection. That course put it all together for me.

I have learned that my genes have nothing to do with me being sick! I can get fully healthy and lose my weight if I just give my body a chance. That brings me to Dr. David Wendel's words, "Stay away from bread, rice, muffins, pizza, waffles, and all packaged foods." He says this every time he sees me in his office. Yup, I see him for chiropractic adjustments to my spine, but he also is super knowledgeable about nutrition and is trained in Applied Kinesiology which tests the strength of various muscles in the body, directly proportional to organ function and overall health and wellness.

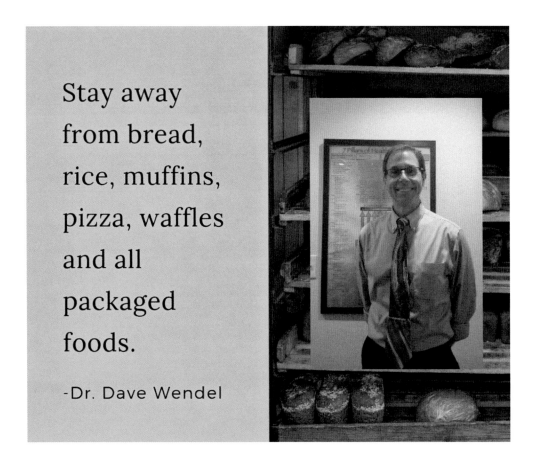

Stay away from bread, rice, muffins, pizza, waffles and all packaged foods.

-Dr. Dave Wendel

Don't get me wrong when I first started with him many years ago, I was very apprehensive. I would say to myself, "How can my arm strength tell this doctor what I should not be ingesting?" Today I am a believer in Applied Kinesiology!

It took about 8 years, lots of learning, and of course trial and error on my part to finally see that what he has been telling me all along is what I should be doing. Easier said than done.

I saw a significant difference from pulling all breads out of my diet, even the ones that are supposedly good for you. I thought that because I was eating brown rice bread or Ezekiel bread it was healthy for me. Well it may be for some, for my body at that time it was not the right thing to do.

I wanted to get off my diabetes medicines and finally cure my body of not only diabetes but all of the ailments I had, especially arthritis. Did you know that arthritis is the beginning stages of pre-diabetes? According to the arthritis foundation, "People with diagnosed diabetes are nearly twice as likely to have arthritis, indicating a diabetes-arthritis connection."

As I mentioned earlier in this book, I was told by my general doctor a few months ago that I can stop all diabetes medicines. I decided to wean myself off of them slowly this time. I monitor my numbers closely. They are steadily stable at 100 - 120 in am. I should be off the last one of them soon.

In the meantime I am working on still tweaking my nutrition and daily exercise. I am diligently working on changing habits that take me backwards and get me off track. Like Dr. George Kosmides always said, "Leave perfection to the tailor."

I continue to listen to my body, breathe, and move forward daily towards my health goals while eating my favorite tasty Greek foods. New recipes are already being tested and on their way into print. Stay tuned for my next books with even more Healthy Greek recipes and some new healthy twists on some American favorites, inspired by my father who owned and cooked in the New Oakland Coffee Shop in Brooklyn, NY for over 30 years.

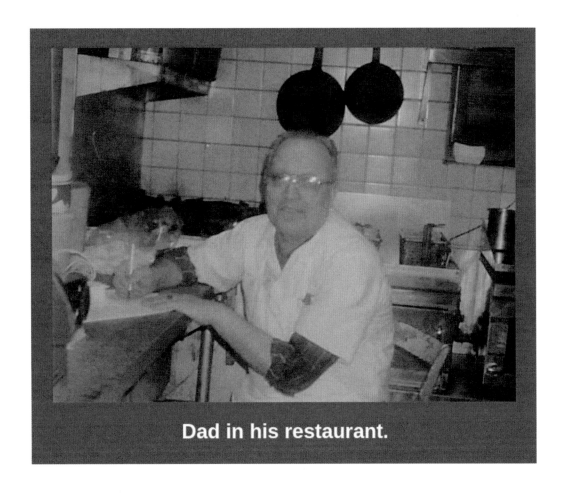

Dad in his restaurant.

Dedication Photo Gallery

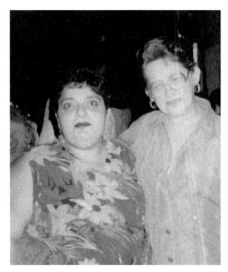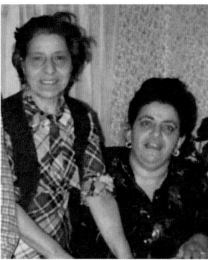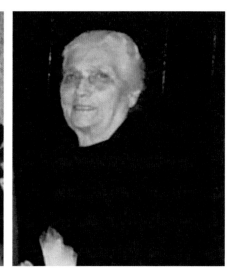

Tina Muller [left] who continued where my mom left off and watched over us like a second mom.

Tina pushed me to start cooking. She taught me to make first pastitsio and not be afraid of cooking. My mother was a perfect cook and taught Tina who is German.

Violet Azarian [middle] gave us love and attention and showed us how to have fun and enjoy every little thing without using money.

Violet taught me to cook American dishes. Her husband was Armenian so she expanded my cooking repertoire beyond Greek and American dishes.

Gia Gia (Grandma) Anna Matheos [right]you watched us every summer and pushed us to be strong, independent women and not take anything lying down.

My grandma was a very strong woman. She had skin cancer and fought until her last breath. I lived with her in Greece. My first husband and I lived in the same building. I visited her every summer with my brother and sister. She had my sister and I scrubbing floors and washing clothes by hand. My brother was a boy so he got to do whatever he wanted including going fishing. I loved her laugh. To get her to laugh took some doing and happened on rare occasions. She was strict and she loved all of us very much.

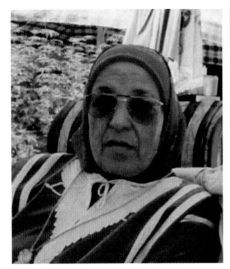 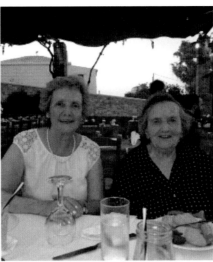 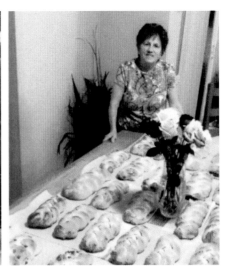

Bahia Mokhtar Attia (my mother-in-law, Essam's mom) [left] I miss your laugh and love of your family. Thank you for showing me what that looks like. I know how hard you worked to keep everyone together. I love you and miss you. I called her Mama Haga. All of her children and grandchildren miss her as well.

Stella Matheos [middle] thank you for sharing your love of cooking and your mom Gia Gia Ermioni Koffinas with me. The kindness and strength that comes out of this woman is just jaw dropping.

Stella is really funny. We laugh quite a bit when we are together. She is my step-mother and my brother Peter's mom. Stella is a perfectionist when it comes to cooking and she is a very good cook.

Nina Sarris [right] thanks for showing me what the words kindness, good heartedness, and strong look like. I love being part of your family and I appreciate you always remembering my son on every holiday and treating him like a grandson.

Nina makes loaves of bread for Easter and Christmas and everyone loves her and her breads. She makes a great spinach pie and an amazing rice pudding. I will be bugging her for her rice pudding recipe for my next book. Right Nina? She has amazing energy and a great laugh. You can just feel the love when you are around her.

Our Family Chefs

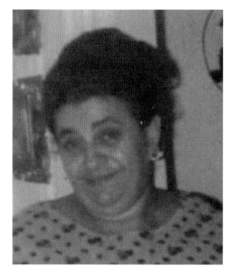

My Mom
Eugenia Matheos

Recipes
Gigantes Ala Eugenia
Eugenia's Avgolemono
Karidopita Ala Eugenia

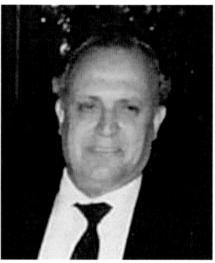

My Dad
Panagiotis Matheos

Recipe
Panagiotis Horta

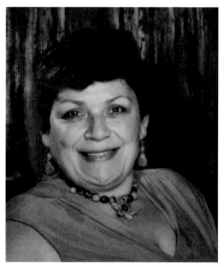

My Sister
Anne P. Matheos

Recipe
Fasolakia Ala Anna

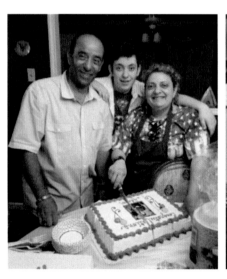

My Husband
Essam Eliraky

Recipe
Stuffed Porgies

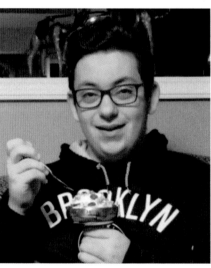

My Son
Adam Eliraky

Recipe
Greek Yogurt Parfait

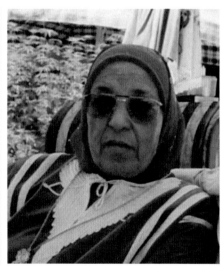

My Mother-In-Law
Bahia Mokhtar Attia

Recipes
Falafel & Karkadea

Our Family Chefs cont.

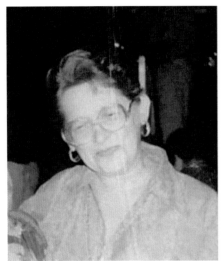

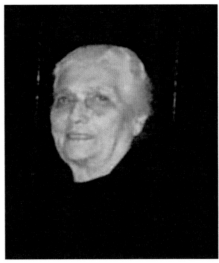

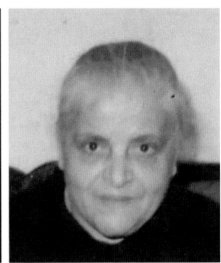

My Aunt Tina
Tina Muller

My Paternal Grandmother
Gia Gia Anna

My Maternal Grandmother
Gia Gia Maria

Recipes
Beets Salad
Pastitsio

Recipes
Chamomile
Lentil Soup

Recipe
Revithia

Heritage and Legacy Photos

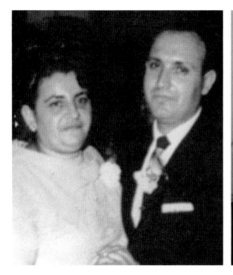 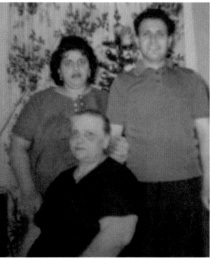 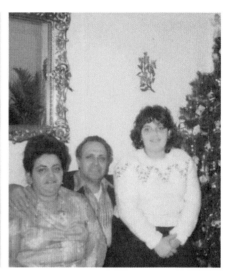

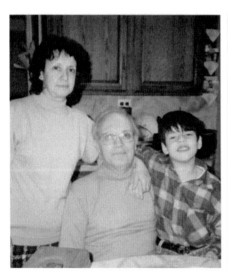 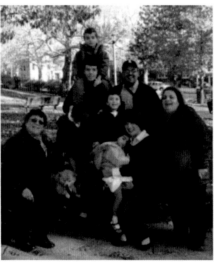 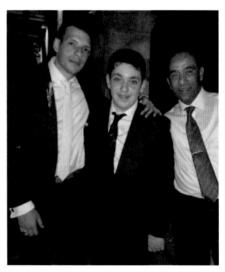

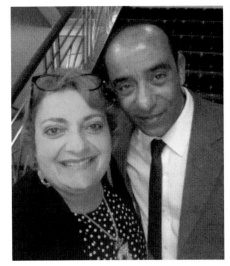 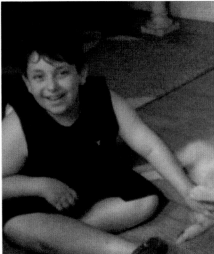 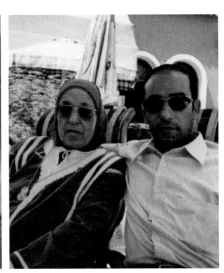

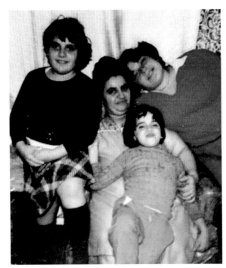 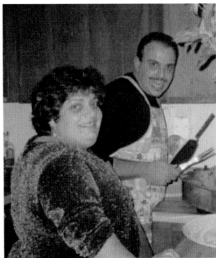 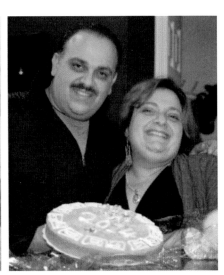

Trips

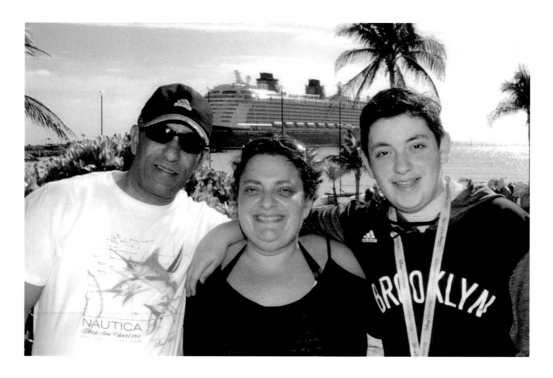

2015 Bahamas

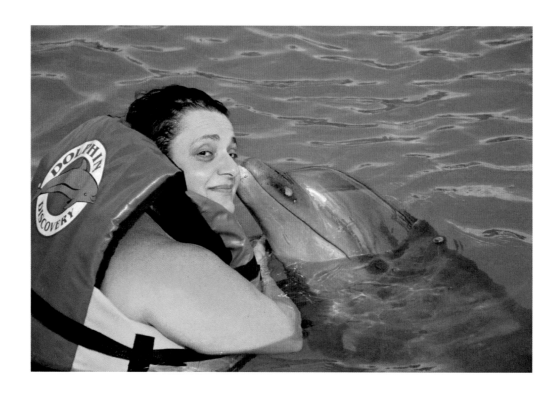

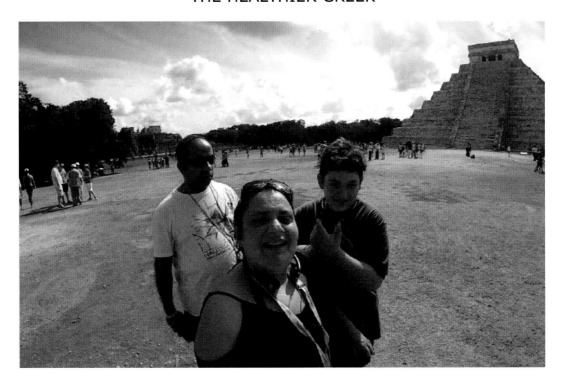

2016 Mexico

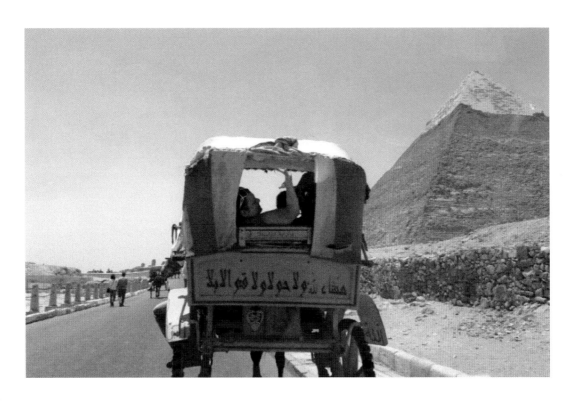

2017 Egypt

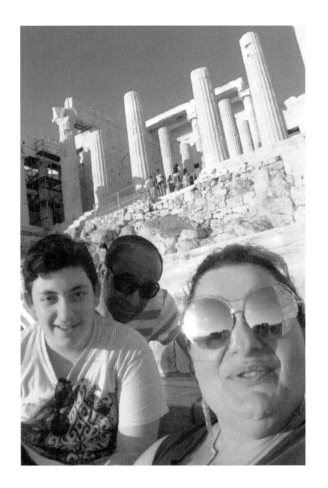

Acropolis in Greece 2017

We walked all the way up to the top of the Acropolis, uneven steps and slippery marble. I was happy to have made it to the top, especially after a full knee replacement. I took a break and we took some pics; it was tough coming back down. I was shaking. I needed to take many breaks on the way down. Once I got home, I vowed to get stronger for the Alaska trip we planned for the following summer.

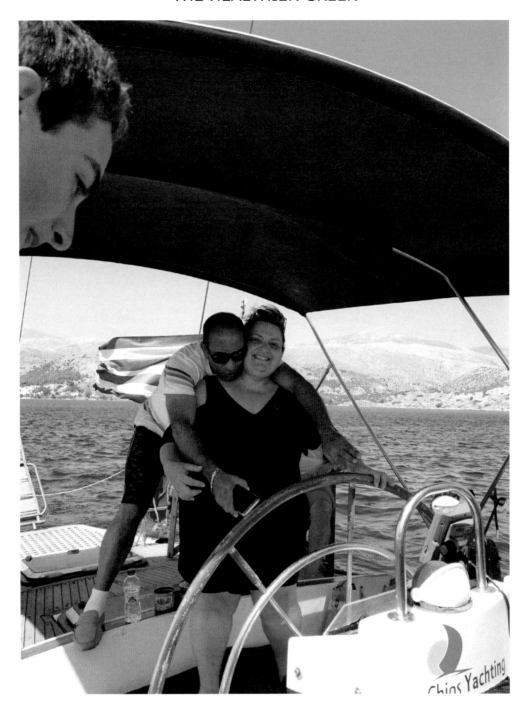

2017 from Egypt to Greece

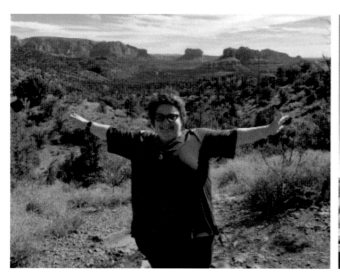 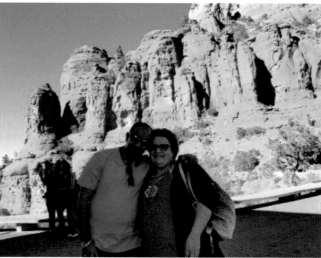

In 2017 we also traveled to Sedona, AZ

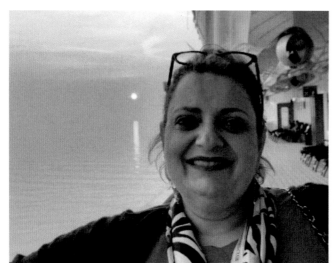 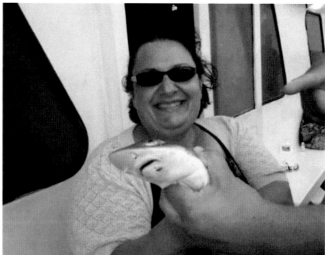

2018 Alaskan Cruise

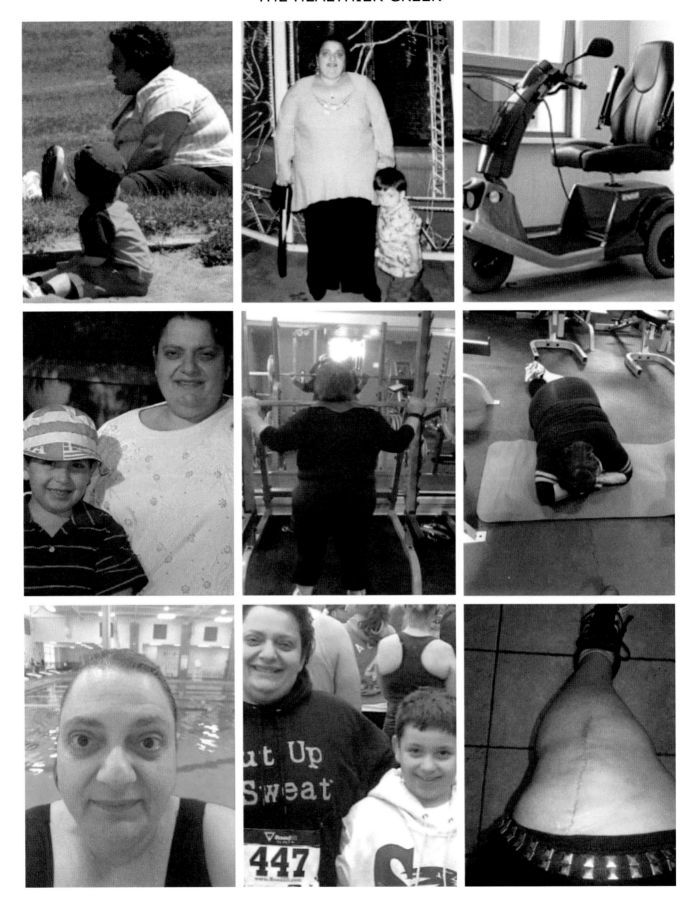

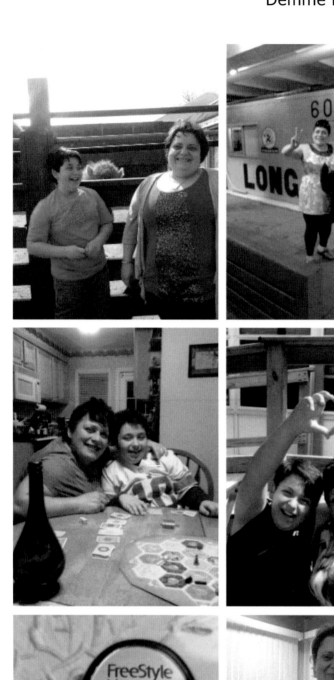
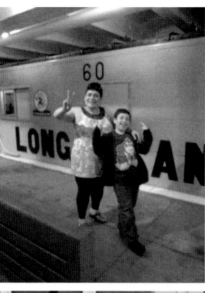
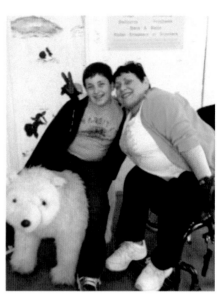
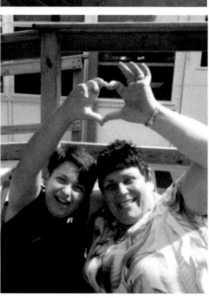
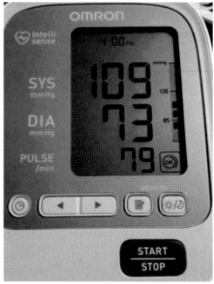
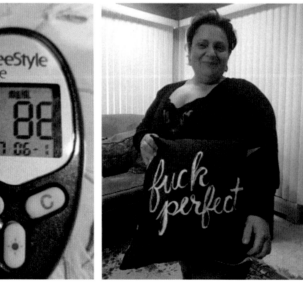
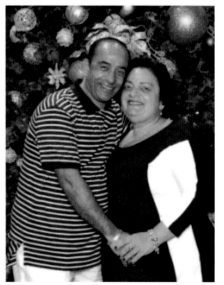

A Note From My Son

Dear Mom,

Without you in my life now I wouldn't be me. You have taught me every essential that I need to live my life to the fullest. You have taught me how to eat healthy and live healthy. You showed me how to be strong even when we feel like we can't be.

By watching you push yourself every day I have learned that even if you are in pain and don't want to go on anymore you should push yourself, not just for yourself but for the loved ones around you as well.

You may not see it, but I try my hardest to be as strong, healthy, and wise as you are every single day of my life. Without you I would be nothing, so thank you for pushing yourself beyond your limit not just for yourself but for me. Thank you for being the greatest mom I could ever ask for.

Love,

Adam

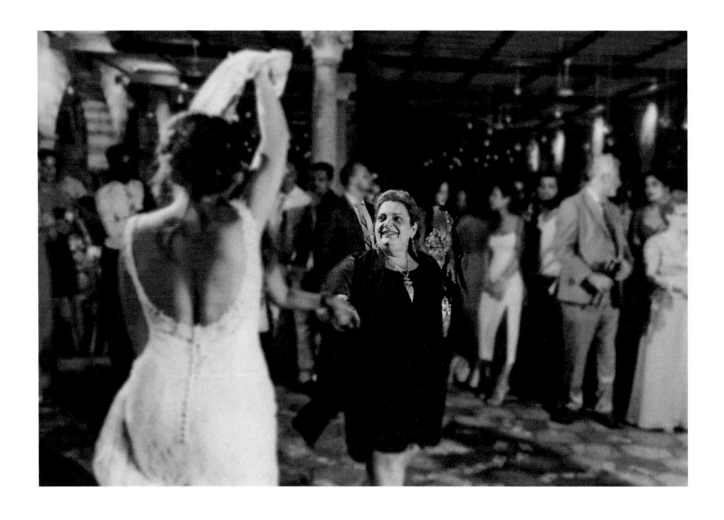

June 2017 Living My Life To The Fullest!!!

Demme Matheos